Atlas of
Obstetric and
Gynecologic
Ultrasound

Atlas of Obstetric and Gynecologic Ultrasound

Dennis A. Sarti, M.D.
Department of Radiology
University of California at Los Angeles
Center for the Health Sciences
Los Angeles, California

With a foreword by
Lawrence D. Platt, M.D.

G. K. Hall Medical Publishers
70 Lincoln Street
Boston, Massachusetts 02111

G. K. Hall Medical Publishers
70 Lincoln Street
Boston, Massachusetts 02111

84 85 86 87 / 4 3 2 1

Sarti, Dennis A.
    Atlas of obstetric and gynecologic ultrasound.

    Includes index.
    1. Ultrasonics in obstetrics.   2. Generative organs,
Female—Diseases—Diagnosis.   3. Diagnosis, Ultrasonic.
I. Title.   [DNLM: 1. Genital diseases, Female—Diagnosis
—Atlases.   2. Pregnancy complications—Diagnosis—
Atlases.   3. Ultrasonics—Diagnostic use—Atlases.
4. Fetal diseases—Diagnosis—Atlases.   WP 17 S249a]
RG527.5.U48S27   1984   618   83-22840
ISBN 0-8161-2262-8

The author and publisher have worked to ensure that all information in this book concerning
drug dosages, schedules, and routes of administration is accurate at the time of publication.
As medical research and practice advance, however, therapeutic standards may change. For
this reason, and because human and mechanical errors will sometimes occur, we recom-
mend that our readers consult the *PDR* or a manufacturer's product information sheet prior to
prescribing or administering any drug discussed in this volume.

Contents

Foreword

Since publication of the first edition of the classic textbook *Diagnostic Ultrasound: Text and Cases* by Dennis A. Sarti and W. Frederick Sample, diagnostic ultrasound has seen a tremendous surge of interest. Improvement in equipment and the incorporation of ultrasound into many diagnostic and therapeutic procedures have led the way for its use by most clinicians today. Underlying all of these developments has been a solid foundation of general ultrasound principles. This text illustrates these time-honored principles as applied to obstetrics and gynecology.

Dr. Sarti has carefully chosen illustrative cases that not only visually but also clinically capture the attention of the reader. The classic format employed in the original textbook has been maintained and affords the reader easy access to the points described in the text. Because of the great interest in ultrasound imaging in the health care of women, we are fortunate that Dr. Sarti has chosen to publish the obstetric and gynecologic cases in a separate volume for specialists in this field. Dr. Sarti is often considered an ultrasonographer's ultrasonographer, and this masterful text further attests to his reputation.

Lawrence D. Platt, M.D.
Department of Obstetrics and
Gynecology
University of Southern California
School of Medicine

Preface

This book is intended for practicing obstetricians, gynecologists, and residents in the specialty who want a fundamental understanding of diagnostic ultrasound and how it fits into their practice. The usefulness of diagnostic ultrasound in obstetrics and gynecology is well established. This noninvasive technique has had great influence on the care of the developing fetus and is used extensively to confirm and characterize pelvic masses that may prove suspicious on examination.

Following the success of *Diagnostic Ultrasound: Text and Cases,* I have been encouraged to incorporate the obstetric and gynecologic portions as the foundation for a new atlas. The cases and their discussions from *Diagnostic Ultrasound* have been reproduced with minor revisions. The text has been rewritten to emphasize what obstetricians and gynecologists can expect from the results of an ultrasound examination, and I have tried to present information that will be helpful in determining whether an ultrasound examination will be useful and appropriate in various clinical settings. Finally, the appendix contains a concise discussion of the physics and techniques of diagnostic ultrasound necessary to successful, high quality scans and correct interpretation.

Most obstetricians and gynecologists have become involved in some way with this imaging modality during the last decade; some perform ultrasound examinations in their offices while others refer patients to sonologists or radiologists. As equipment has improved and diagnoses have become more sophisticated, the need has grown for information to supplement the knowledge gained from short courses in ultrasonography. I hope that this atlas will prove a valuable and useful resource in meeting that need.

Dennis A. Sarti, M.D.

Obstetric Application of Ultrasound

Techniques of Scanning

Obstetric ultrasound had its beginnings in the late 1950s and early 1960s (Donald, MacVicar, and Brown 1958; Donald and Brown 1961). By today's standards, equipment was primitive; present-day studies are quite sophisticated and are almost equivalent to a physical examination of the fetus. Earlier studies used a 1.6- or 2.25-MHz transducer. Today 3.5- or 5.0-MHz transducers are in use. This increase in transducer frequency has resulted in dramatically improved resolution.

Formerly, static B-scan images were preferred over real-time ultrasound because of better resolution. Recent technical improvements have resulted in real-time images equal to those produced by B-scans. Since real-time scanning produces a more thorough examination in a shorter time, it is the procedure of choice if high-quality equipment is used.

A filled urinary bladder is necessary for best scanning results. It provides an ultrasonic window by displacing air-filled bowel out of the pelvis, thus allowing better visualization of the lower uterine segment. An acoustic couplant is necessary between the skin and transducer to eliminate any air interposed between the two. Mineral oil or acoustic gel are the most commonly used materials. Inadequate application of acoustic couplant will lead to poor quality scans and interpretative errors. Inadequate couplant causes a drop-off, with poor registration of weaker echoes, which can make solid masses appear echo free and be misinterpreted as cystic structures.

A specular reflector, which is an anatomic boundary with a large smooth surface (see Appendix), must be scanned at an angle appropriate for accurate visualization. The sound beam should strike such reflectors as close to the perpendicular as possible, as exemplified by visualization of the endocervical canal, especially near the internal os. It is essential to see the internal os when attempting to rule out a placenta previa. If the scan is not made close to the perpendicular of the endocervical canal, it will not be visualized. This often is a problem when scanning with the linear array real-time transducer that is commonly used in obstetric practice. Because of its length and the necessity for adequate skin contact, a linear array transducer often is unable to visualize the endocervical canal. Difficulty in visualizing the internal os often leads to an incorrect diagnosis of placenta previa, when the image actually represents a low-lying placenta. A small-sector real-time scanner will supply a more accurate image of this area.

Ultrasonic Determination of Gestational Age

Since diagnostic ultrasound does not suffer from the magnification distortion produced by x-rays, accurate measurements of anatomic structures can be made. Four such structures measured to determine gestational age include uterine size, gestational sac, crown–rump length, and biparietal diameter. Use of ultrasound to resolve discrepancies between menstrual history and uterine size is discussed later in this chapter.

Uterine size is continually evaluated during pregnancy by the obstetrician, so that the ultrasonographer often prefers to measure other anatomic structures that are more accurate. The gestation sac is measured from the fifth to tenth menstrual week. Most accurate measurements of gestational age come from evaluation of the crown–rump length, which is used from the sixth to the fourteenth week. The most commonly measured structure for gestational age is the biparietal diameter (Campbell 1969; Flamme 1972; Levi 1971), which is measured from 12 weeks until term and is least accurate near term.

Before delving into the ultrasonic findings of dating a pregnancy, discussion of pertinent anatomy is in order. Several ovarian follicles begin to mature and ripen at the same time with usually only one rupturing and entering the distal fallopian tube. The remaining, less ripened follicles undergo atresia. The ovum is transported down the tube via ciliary action and muscular contraction. It takes approximately 3–4 days to traverse the tube and enter the uterus. If fertilization fails to occur, the corpus luteum begins to decrease in size approximately 9 days after ovulation. This decreases the progesterone level and eventually causes menstrual bleeding 14 days after ovulation (Langman 1969). Without fertilization, the oocyte becomes nonviable within 1–2 days.

Fertilization usually occurs in the ampullary end of the fallopian tube. The corpus luteum increases in size and remains functionally active through the first half of pregnancy; it secretes progesterone, so menstruation does not occur. During the 3–4 days needed to traverse the tube, the fertilized ovum increases to the 8- to 16-cell stage. It has a mulberry appearance and is called a morula. As the morula enters the uterine cavity, fluid begins to accumulate centrally, and a blastocyst is formed. This floats within the uterine cavity until it finally attaches to the endometrium around the sixth day after fertilization. Trophoblastic cells begin to penetrate the epithelial cells of the uterine mucosa due to the production of proteolytic enzymes by the trophoblast. By the eleventh to twelfth day, the blastocyst is completely embedded within the endometrial stroma. The decidua is fairly even over the entire blastocyst along with the developing villous system. The decidua basalis is that area in contact with the chorion frondosum which eventually develops into the placenta. This area has an excellent blood supply and gives rise to high-level echoes on ultrasound. The decidua capsularis is in contact with the chorion laeve, which is also highly echogenic early in pregnancy.

As gestation advances, and the blastocyst enlarges, however, the blood supply of the expanding decidua capsularis decreases, and the villous system, which is the chorion laeve, atrophies and disappears. The chorion frondosum maintains abundant blood supply, proliferates, and develops into a placenta. It is at this stage, at approximately 10–11 menstrual weeks, that the gestation sac "disappears" due to the decreasing blood supply of the stretched and enlarging decidua capsularis and the eventual atrophy of the chorion laeve.

While the gestational sac is primarily fluid-filled, the embryo is growing rapidly. The following table (Langman 1969) indicates the crown–rump length compared to the weeks since fertilization.

Weeks since fertilization	Crown–rump length
5	5–8 mm
6	10–14 mm
7	17–22 mm
8	28–30 mm

At the sixth or seventh week after menstruation, the embryo finally obtains a size large enough to be detected by ultrasound. Prior to this, only the highly echogenic chorionic villi of the gestation sac can be visualized.

Normal Gestational Sac

Ultrasonic visualization of the gestational sac first occurs around the fourth to fifth menstrual week. By this time, the blastocyst has implanted itself in the endometrium and is completely surrounded by highly echogenic, vascular chorionic villi. The blastocyst enlarges to 5 or 10 mm and is finally detected. A gestational sac has a circular to oval shape, and its borders are intact. The size of the gestational sac increases rapidly from the fourth to the tenth menstrual week, enlarging from one to approximately 6 cm in mean gestational sac diameter (Gottesfeld 1970). This rapid growth rate gives rise to the accurate dating of pregnancy (Garrett, Grunwald, and Robinson 1970; Gottesfeld 1970). Follow-up examination 7–10 days after an initial study will normally demonstrate a measurable increase in the gestational sac of approximately 7–10 mm. A repeat examination showing appropriate growth is the most accurate and reliable means of determining a viable pregnancy. The majority of gestational sacs are situated in the fundal or miduterine segments. A small percentage have a low implantation site, which can be normal or may lead to placenta previa or abortion (Donald 1969; Garrett, Grunwald, and Robinson 1970; Horger, Kreutner, and Underwood 1974).

Since highly vascular chorionic villi initially surround the sac in its entirety, a high-level echo arises from the gestational sac which is two to three shades of gray darker than surrounding myometrium. This high-level echogenicity is extremely important in evaluating viability, since it documents a healthy surrounding vascular supply. By the tenth menstrual week, the echoes from chorionic villi in contact with the decidua capsularis begin to weaken due to atrophy of the vascular supply, and the gestational sac "disappears." Echoes arising from the embryo within the gestational sac can be seen about the seventh menstrual week when the embryo is approximately 5 mm in size. Fetal cardiac activity can also be detected at this time (Robinson 1972).

Single as well as multiple gestational sacs may be detected in utero. Recent reports have indicated a much higher incidence of twins conceived than are delivered (Robinson and Caines 1977). Multiple gestational sacs, however, may also indicate an impending abortion and follow-up studies are necessary.

Abnormal Gestational Sac

When a patient presents with bleeding in early pregnancy, ultrasound is most helpful in predicting the progress of the pregnancy. If a normal gestational sac and an embryo with cardiac activity are identified, the patient can be assured that a viable pregnancy is present. Conversely, ultrasound findings may indicate an abnormal pregnancy.

Several signs have been described which indicate possible abnormality of the gestational sac. These include: (1) pointed segment, (2) single break or fragmentation, (3) lack of growth, (4) weak surrounding echoes, (5) lack of fetal echoes by the seventh to eighth week, (6) low implantation, and (7) double sac. Several of the above findings are indicative of a nonviable pregnancy while others are only suggestive. As mentioned earlier, the shape of a gestational sac is usually circular to oval. A pointed segment often signals difficulty with the pregnancy if no adjacent masses are present. Distortion of a gestational sac may be caused by uterine myomas or other masses. If the sac has a sharply pointed segment with no identifiable adjacent mass, however, fragmentation or a single break often follows (Donald, Morley, and Barnett 1972; Donald 1969; Hellman et al. 1969). Before diagnosing a break or fragmentation, care must be taken to rule out technical artifacts. If an artifact is not present, these findings are then indicative of a nonviable pregnancy.

The third and probably most important finding of an abnormal gestational sac is lack of adequate growth. If there is any question as to the viability of a pregnancy, the patient should be reexamined in 1 week to 10 days. In this period of time, the sac should enlarge approximately 1 cm in diameter. Lack of growth or decrease in size confirms a nonviable pregnancy (Donald, Morley, and Barnett 1972; Donald 1969; Hellman et al. 1969; Robinson and Caines 1977).

High-level echoes arising from the vascularity of the chorionic villi are evidence of a healthy blood supply to the developing embryo and sac. Therefore, weak surrounding sac echoes, which may be the only sign, are extremely important in diagnosing a nonviable pregnancy. Echoes surrounding the gestational sac are of a higher amplitude than the adjacent myometrium. Normally, there is a decrease in echogenicity of the chorionic villi in contact with the decidua capsularis at approximately the tenth or eleventh menstrual week. This is due to atrophy of the chorionic villi as they outgrow their blood supply. The chorion frondosum, which becomes placenta, maintains its high-level echogenicity. Therefore, a pregnancy that is in difficulty and has its blood supply interrupted or decreased will manifest weak surrounding echoes. This finding is most easily detected from the fifth to ninth menstrual week when the surrounding echoes are normally uniform in thickness and amplitude. However, by the tenth or eleventh menstrual week, the gestational sac has "disappeared" secondary to normal vascular atrophy. This normal event should not be misinterpreted as evidence of a nonviable pregnancy.

As noted in the previous discussion of normal anatomy, the embryo attains a size of 5 mm by the seventh menstrual week. By the seventh menstrual week, echoes arising from the embryo should be noted within the gestational sac. Cardiac activity can also be detected by real time or Doppler. An anembryonic pregnancy should be detected by the eighth or ninth menstrual week, when a definite diagnosis of a nonviable pregnancy can be reached.

The last two signs of possible gestational sac abnormality, low implantation and double sac, are only suggestive of abnormality and must be reevaluated by a later ultrasound examination. There are conflicting reports as to the implication of a low implantation site. The usual implantation site is fundal or mid uterine. Several investigators have reported an increased incidence of abortion with low implantation (Donald, Morley, and Barnett 1972; Donald 1969; Hellman et al. 1969). Others have found no increased incidence of abortion unless bleeding is clinically evident (Garrett, Grunwald, and Robinson 1970; Kohorn and Kaufman 1974). The safest course to follow with a low implantation pregnancy is a repeat examination one to two weeks later to evaluate the progression of the pregnancy. A low implantation is felt by some investigators to lead to placenta previa (Horger, Kreutner, and Underwood 1974), but this is disputed by others and further studies are necessary to answer the question (Kohorn and Kaufman 1974). Double gestational sac is the final sign which can be indicative of an impending abortion (Garrett, Grunwald, and Robinson 1970; Hellman et al. 1969; Robinson and Caines 1977). Doubling of the gestation sac may indicate a twin gestation, but it may also indicate an abnormal pregnancy and a follow-up examination in 7–10 days is indicated.

Crown–Rump Length

The most accurate ultrasonic determination of gestational age is measurement of crown–rump length. The embryo is a rapidly growing structure at this stage and increases in size from a few millimeters to 8 cm from the sixth to fourteenth menstrual weeks. An important factor in obtaining an accurate crown–rump length is correctly determining the long axis of the embryo. The embryo is very active at this stage of pregnancy, and correctly aligning the transducer may be difficult. This has become an easier task with real-time scanners. While determining the crown–rump length, fetal cardiac activity can be documented. Major anomalies such as anencephaly may be detected at this time.

Biparietal Diameter

From 14 weeks until term the biparietal diameter is measured to provide an estimate of gestational age. The biparietal diameter can be seen as early as the twelfth menstrual week and should be seen in nearly all cases by the fifteenth to sixteenth week, except where there are unusual technical difficulties (Leopold and Asher 1975).

The growth rate of the biparietal diameter is more rapid early in pregnancy. From approximately 15 to 30 weeks, it grows at 3 mm per week; from 30 weeks to term the growth rate drops to 1 to 2 mm per week (Gottesfeld 1975). Because of this normal variation in growth rate, a measurement of biparietal diameter early in pregnancy is much more accurate in estimating gestation than one taken later in pregnancy. Regrettably, many patients are sent for their first ultrasound examination at 35 weeks, when accuracy at estimating gestation is poorest. If a patient is at risk for a troublesome pregnancy, it is best to order an ultrasound examination as early in the pregnancy as possible. A follow-up study later in pregnancy is of great assistance in clinical assessment of suspected intrauterine growth retardation.

The correct technique for determining biparietal diameter is critical to obtain accurate, reproducible measurements. Longitudinal scans of the uterus are performed initially to visualize the orientation and position of the fetus and fetal skull. While scanning the fetal skull, attempts are made to visualize the falx cerebri by varying the transducer angle. Since the falx is a specular reflector, the sound beam must strike close to the perpendicular for it to be visualized. The angle of the transducer necessary to visualize the falx is called the *angle of ascynclitism.* Once the angle of ascynclitism has been determined, transverse scans of the fetal skull are obtained using the correct angulation. If the correct angle is not used, the falx may not be visualized and the skull will have an unusual configuration. Repeat scans are performed from the base of the skull to the top until the thalami come into view. The thalami appear as two triangular lucencies on each side of the midline. Several scans are produced at this site to check accuracy. The biparietal diameter is measured at this level and represents the distance between the skull echoes. Since ultrasound does not suffer from the magnification artifacts produced by x-ray, direct measurements are reported.

Several common technical difficulties can arise. Measurements often are taken too cephalad on the fetal skull. On such scans, the falx is seen to course the entire length, separating the cerebral hemispheres. Measurements reported at this higher level will be too small, and gestational age will be interpreted less than actual (Brown 1975). It is necessary to scan more caudad on the fetal skull until there is some disruption of the falx and the thalami come into view.

Gray-scale ultrasound is the cause of another common source of measurement error. The echoes of the fetal head include skull, muscle, subcutaneous tissue, skin, and hair. Deciding where to measure may lead to a discrepancy of several millimeters. Skull echoes are best seen when output and sensitivity are decreased on the ultrasound units. Once the correct scanning plane is determined, output and sensitivity should be decreased to enhance visualization of the skull echoes. A biparietal diameter then can be accurately measured.

Even the most careful laboratory procedures may result in a 1- to 2-mm error. Remember that later in pregnancy the growth rate of biparietal diameter is 1 to 2 mm per week, thus requiring great care and meticulous scanning technique in biparietal diameter determinations. An accurate measurement of biparietal diameter is possible in the vast majority of patients. There is, however, a small number (2% to 3%) in whom this determination is not possible technically. This usually is due to the position and angulation of the fetal head. In such instances, measurements of the fetal abdomen and fetal femur will give an approximation of gestational age.

Bleeding in the First Trimester

Bleeding in the first trimester is a common clinical entity. The causes of first trimester bleeding are varied, and some can be diagnosed by ultrasound. These include placental position, impending abortion, necrotic fibroids, cervical abnormalities, and ectopic pregnancy.

As discussed earlier in this chapter, a normal gestation sac is seen from the fifth to tenth menstrual week. By the eighth or ninth week, the gestation sac will have thicker echoes on one side, indicating placental position (Ghorashi and Gottesfeld 1977). Diagnostic ultrasound accurately locates placental position (Gottesfeld, Thompson, Holmes, and Taylor 1966; Sanders and Conrad 1975). The ultrasonic appearance depends on what is situated between the transducer and the placenta. An anterior placenta has an even parenchymal pattern described as speckled in appearance. The chorionic plate is a sharp linear echo covering the placenta. Since it is a specular reflector, the chorionic plate is visualized only when the sound beam strikes it close to the perpendicular of its surface. A posterior placenta also has a speckled appearance when it is situated behind amniotic fluid. Since fluid minimally attenuates sound, the weak parenchymal echoes reflected back from the placenta are able to reach the transducer. If the fetus is anterior to the placenta, the weak placental parenchymal echoes are attenuated by the fetus. Therefore, a posterior placenta will have an echo-free appearance behind the fetus and a speckled appearance behind amniotic fluid. This often leads to confusion in determining the boundaries of a posterior placenta.

Uterine size enlarges at a more rapid rate than does the placenta during pregnancy. The end result is that proportionally less surface area of the uterine cavity is covered by placenta later in pregnancy compared to earlier stages (Sanders and Conrad 1975). This phenomenon is one explanation for false diagnosis of placenta previa early in pregnancy. Bleeding that occurs from 13 to 16 menstrual weeks often is secondary to low placental position. As the uterus enlarges it pulls the placenta away from the internal os and lower uterine segment. This may lead to slight separation of the distal placenta with bleeding, which may appear on ultrasound and be seen near the placental caudad border. The placenta moves further away from the internal os as the uterus enlarges during the remainder of pregnancy. These patients often continue their pregnancy without any further episodes of bleeding.

First-trimester bleeding may indicate an impending abortion. The ultrasonic findings of an abnormal gestation sac have been discussed. The main function of ultrasound in a threatened abortion is to document fetal viability. Failure to identify fetal cardiac activity indicates that the embryo is too small for cardiac activity to be detected or that the pregnancy is not viable. Once the embryo reaches a crown–rump length of 1.0 to 1.5 cm, fetal cardiac activity usually is detectable with present-day equipment. It is better to err on the safe side, however, and to conduct a repeat exam in 7 to 10 days. At that time the crown–rump length should be 2.0 to 2.5 cm, and cardiac activity should be readily apparent.

Ectopic pregnancy is a cause of first-trimester bleeding and is discussed separately later in this chapter.

Bleeding in the Third Trimester

Third-trimester bleeding may be secondary to two major complications of pregnancy: placenta previa and placenta abruptio. Ultrasound is helpful in the diagnosis of these entities, especially placenta previa.

Adequate urinary bladder filling is necessary for the diagnosis of placenta previa. If the urinary bladder is not well distended, the lower uterine segment and cervix are collapsed and the internal os cannot be seen. On the other hand, the urinary bladder may be overfilled, pressing together the anterior and posterior components of the lower uterine segment. This leads to a false impression of the internal os situated more cephalad than is true. Urinary bladder filling must be sufficient to stretch out the cervix and lower uterus without overdistending the bladder to the point of compressing the lower uterine segment.

The internal cervical os should be visualized in order to determine if a placenta previa is present. First, the axis of the cervix is found. Most often the cervix will be midline and parallel to the central axis of the body; however, the cervical axis may be off center and angled to the right or left. This is easily noted on transverse scans of the cervix and lower uterine segment. Serial longitudinal scans parallel to the long axis of the cervix are obtained at 2- to 3-mm intervals until the linear echo of the endocervical canal comes into view. At this point the internal os can be visualized. This scanning technique for evaluating the endocervical canal is easily and quickly performed and is most helpful in diagnosing clinical entities such as placenta previa and incompetent cervix (Sarti, Sample, Hobel, and Staisch 1979).

Placental position is relatively consistent from one study to another, although uterine contractions and varying urinary bladder filling may rotate the uterus. This occasionally causes the placenta to appear in a different position than noted on a previous study. If a contraction is present in the lower uterine segments, it draws the placenta closer to the internal os and produces the appearance of a placenta previa. It may be necessary to wait for the contraction to relax for the true relationship between the inferior border of the placenta and the internal os to be evaluated.

A low-lying placenta or possible placenta previa commonly is suspected early in pregnancy, or from 12 to 16 weeks. In the great majority of these cases, a study later in pregnancy will indicate no evidence of a placenta previa. The enlarging uterus pulls the placenta further away from the internal os, so that a low-lying placenta or questionable previa early in pregnancy very often is well removed from the cervix near term. When placenta previa is diagnosed later in pregnancy, around 35 weeks, it usually will persist in that position until term.

An anterior placenta previa is easily diagnosed by ultrasound. Since the parenchymal echoes return to the transducer, the boundary of an anterior placenta usually is visualized in its entirety. This is not true for a posterior placenta. Since the fetus attenuates the weak parenchymal echoes as they return, the entire boundary of a posterior placenta may not be visualized. A posterior placenta previa often is a difficult diagnosis. There are certain clues in an ultrasound examination that should raise the index of suspicion and that warrant closer scrutiny of the internal os.

When the fetus is in a cephalic position, the distance between the maternal sacrum and the fetal cranium should be noted. If this distance is less than 15 mm, a low-lying placenta or posterior placenta previa usually is excluded (King 1973). If this distance is greater than 15 mm, the possibility of a posterior placenta previa exists, and attempts should be made to visualize the internal os. By manipulating the fetus and elevating the fetal head slightly out of the pelvis, a small amount of amniotic fluid can be visualized adjacent to the internal os. If this has a sharp V-shaped appearance and is surrounded by myometrium, a posterior placenta previa can be excluded. If placental tissue is noted in the region, a placenta previa is present. By elevating the fetal head, amniotic fluid will provide an excellent ultrasonic window for better visualization of the lower uterine segment and internal os.

There are causes other than a posterior placenta previa that may elevate the fetal cranial echoes off the maternal sacrum. If an extremity is situated posterior to the fetal skull, the distance between the maternal sacrum and fetal skull is increased. Other causes include the cervix not in midline with the internal os displaced to the right or left and the fetal skull positioned off center. Therefore, a fetal skull to maternal sacrum distance greater than 15 mm is not diagnostic of a posterior placenta previa, but it definitely requires closer inspection of the area. Another clue suggestive of placenta previa is a fetus in an unusual lie. A breech, transverse, or oblique lie should always raise the suspicion of a placenta previa.

The second major cause of third-trimester bleeding that can be diagnosed by ultrasound is abruptio placenta. Abruptio placenta is less common than placenta previa and often is of such an emergent nature that the patient is brought straight to the operating room rather than waiting for an examination. It is a more difficult ultrasonic diagnosis than a placenta previa. An initial clue may be visualization of fluid in the vagina secondary to hemorrhage. Examination of the placental myometrial interface often shows a large lucency separating the two structures. This is secondary to hemorrhage in the area. The novice ultrasonographer may often misinterpret a normal finding as an abruptio placenta. Prominent tubular vessels normally are present between the placenta and myometrium. In some patients this lush vascular region may appear as a large lucent area, suggesting an abruptio placenta.

The ultrasonic findings of abruptio placenta include an abnormally located lucent area suggestive of hemorrhage. This may be located between the placenta and myometrium or within the amniotic sac. The placenta often has an abnormal contour relative to the myometrium as though being separated from it. If such findings are present in the appropriate clinical setting, then an abruptio placenta may be diagnosed.

As term approaches, the placenta becomes more mature. Areas of hemorrhage may arise inside the placenta, and the cotyledons can appear very lucent. It is important that these normal sonolucent-areas, which arise secondary to placental maturation, are not diagnosed as abruptio placenta (Winsberg 1973).

Size-Dates Discrepancy

In early pregnancy the patient's menstrual history is compared clinically to uterine size. Most often there is good correlation, and the last menstrual period is used as the clinical gauge for dating the pregnancy. Not infrequently, there is a discrepancy between the palpable uterine size and menstrual history. When the uterine size and menstrual history do not correspond, an ultrasound examination often is used to resolve the discrepancy.

As noted earlier, ultrasonic dating of pregnancy depends upon measuring the size of specific anatomic structures such as the gestational sac, crown–rump length, and biparietal diameter. Ultrasonic dating is most accurate in early pregnancy, and discrepancy with menstrual history will be readily apparent.

The uterus and its contents may be larger or smaller than expected from the menstrual history. If smaller, the most common causes are incorrect dates or an abortion in progress. Ultrasonic signs of an abortion have already been discussed. Many more causes are present when the palpable uterine size is larger than expected from the menstrual history. Ultrasound provides specific answers to this dilemma. Some of the causes for larger size than dates would indicate include incorrect dates, multiple gestation, polyhydramnios, hydatidiform mole, and a pelvic mass in conjunction with pregnancy. Diagnosing these various etiologies will not only correctly date the pregnancy but also will explain the cause of the size-dates discrepancy.

Incorrect Dates

The most common cause of disparity between clinical assessment of uterine size and menstrual history is confusion in determining the last menstrual period. The patient's menstrual cycle may be variable, or she may not recall the date of her last period. Spotting in early pregnancy often is misinterpreted as menses. When such instances arise, an early ultrasound examination can clarify the situation. Since ultrasonic dating is most accurate early in pregnancy with measurement of the gestational sac or crown–rump length, establishing a correct date for the last menstrual period is best achieved at that time. If there is confusion and the obstetrician waits until later in the pregnancy for clarification, ultrasonic dating is less accurate and may not resolve the problem.

Multiple Gestation

A multiple gestation increases uterine size and is a common cause of size greater than dates would indicate. An ultrasound examination easily identifies multiple gestation. Twins can be diagnosed as early as 5 to 6 menstrual weeks with visualization of a double gestational sac (Levi 1976). Since there are other causes of a double gestational sac, twins cannot be diagnosed with certainty until both embryos are visualized. The embryos become large enough to be detected by the seventh menstrual week.

If bleeding is present, a double gestational sac may be a sign of impending abortion. There are reports that a greater number of twins are diagnosed early in pregnancy than are delivered at term (Hellman, Kobayashi, and Cromb 1973; Levi 1976). This finding may be secondary to a twin gestation with one viable pregnancy and one blighted ovum. Because of these factors, visualization of a double gestational sac raises the possibility of a twin gestation, but the diagnosis cannot be made until both embryos are visualized. The other possibilities should be kept in mind, and a study at a later date may be necessary to confirm multiple gestation.

When a multiple gestation is identified, care must be taken to determine the correct number. Triplets often are misdiagnosed as twins. This was a common error when only a B-scanning technique was used. Real-time examination decreases this diagnostic error. It is important to develop a three-dimensional concept of the uterine contents so that triplets will not be missed. Quintuplets have been diagnosed as early as 9 menstrual weeks (Campbell and Dewhurst 1970).

There has been some dispute as to the biparietal diameter growth ratio in a multiple gestation. It has been shown that the growth rate of the biparietal diameter in twin and single pregnancies are similar (Scheer 1974).

Ultrasonic evaluation also is exceedingly helpful when amniocentesis is performed in a multiple gestation. The location of the separate amniotic sacs are identified, and appropriate puncture sites are determined. Such information assures the withdrawal of fluid from the separate cavities.

Polyhydramnios

Another cause for uterine size larger than indicated by menstrual dates is polyhydramnios. Increased amniotic fluid increases uterine volume and may cause excessive uterine enlargement. Ultrasonic evaluation of amniotic fluid volume is difficult and requires years of experience. At present, there is no accurate, quantitative means for determining amniotic fluid volume by ultrasound examination. It remains a qualitative judgment by the ultrasonographer. Analysis of only one or two scans often leads to a mistaken impression of polyhydramnios. A three-dimensional conceptualization of uterine contents is required of the individual performing the examination. A very active fetus that moves to different regions in the uterine cavity can result in misinterpretation of polyhydramnios. Best results are obtained by rapidly scanning the uterine cavity with real-time ultrasound to obtain a quick, accurate, three-dimensional assessment of amniotic fluid volume.

It is important to note that there is a normal variation in the proportion between amniotic fluid and fetal volume during the course of pregnancy. In early pregnancy, from approximately 10 to 26 weeks, there appears to be a relatively increased amount of amniotic fluid compared to fetal volume. After 35 weeks the opposite is true; it then appears that a relatively decreased amount of fluid is present. Appreciation of this normal variation in relative amniotic fluid volume during the progression of pregnancy is necessary for an accurate assessment of polyhydramnios.

Polyhydramnios usually is of unknown etiology. Since amniotic fluid is turned over so rapidly, a slight imbalance between mother and fetus can lead to polyhydramnios. Close scrutiny of the fetus under these circumstances will demonstrate no abnormalities.

In the presence of polyhydramnios, the ultrasonographer should concentrate the examination on certain areas of the fetus. Polyhydramnios often is an indicator of obstruction to the fetal gastrointestinal tract or other difficulties of fetal swallowing. Close scrutiny of the fetal gastrointestinal tract can lead to the diagnosis of such entities as esophageal, duodenal, and jejunal atresia. Evaluation of the fetal thorax and abdomen demonstrates abnormal fluid collections, which leads to a diagnosis of gastrointestinal obstruction. The level and location of the various fluid collections often determines the type of obstruction that is present. Detection of these fluid areas will explain the initial finding of polyhydramnios.

Anencephaly is another cause of polyhydramnios and should immediately come to mind in the presence of too much fluid. Since biparietal diameter measurements can be obtained in 100% of cases by 15 weeks, a diagnosis of anencephaly easily is made by this time of pregnancy.

Finally, polyhydramnios is seen in fetal demise. The amount of amniotic fluid present in cases of fetal demise is variable and ranges from severe oligohydramnios to severe polyhydramnios.

Hydatidiform Mole

Hydatidiform mole is another cause of size-dates discrepancy during pregnancy. The uterus reaches 16-week size without any detectable fetal heart tones. The patient often experiences hyperemesis and some vaginal spotting. These symptoms prompt ultrasound evaluation of the uterus. Before the advent of ultrasonography, the diagnosis of a hydatidiform mole was difficult. The ultrasonic appearance of a hydatidiform mole is so characteristic that the diagnosis now is easy and rapid. Examination of the uterus demonstrates a diffuse, even, speckled appearance throughout, suggesting only placental type echoes (Leopold 1971; Sanders and Conrad 1975; Thompson 1973). There is no evidence of the strong, high-amplitude fetal echoes.

Theca-lutein cysts often are present in conjunction with a molar pregnancy secondary to the markedly elevated human chorionic gonadotropin levels. These cysts appear as large, multiloculated, bilateral cystic masses and confirm a molar pregnancy. Although the ultrasonic appearance of a hydatidiform mole is very characteristic, there are several entities that may give a similar ultrasonic appearance. These include (1) severely degenerating pregnancy, (2) degenerating fibroid, and (3) chronic ectopic pregnancy. It should be noted, however, that clinical history and human chorionic gonadotropin levels usually are able to distinguish these from a hydatidiform mole. A small percentage of molar pregnancies are malignant (choriocarcinoma). Ultrasound cannot distinguish between a hydatidiform mole and a choriocarcinoma; therefore, each case of molar pregnancy diagnosed by ultrasound should be treated as a potential choriocarcinoma.

Uterine or Pelvic Mass Plus Pregnancy

When a uterine or pelvic mass is present in addition to pregnancy, uterine size may appear larger than expected from menstrual history. Masses often elevate the fundus of the uterus in a cephalad direction, which leads to false interpretation of fundal height.

The most common mass arising from the uterus is a fibroid. The ultrasonographic appearance of a uterine myoma usually is characteristic. This homogeneous muscle mass has relatively low-level echoes and increased attenuation compared to normal uterine myometrium. Occasionally, they can be difficult to distinguish from areas of uterine contraction. Fibroids large enough to cause size-dates discrepancy usually are readily identifiable. Many large fibroids undergo degeneration and necrosis. In these instances the ultrasonic presentation will be different. Necrotic areas appear as fluid regions with thick irregular borders. They are differentiated from uncomplicated myomas because of enhanced through transmission present deep to the necrotic areas.

The size and position of the myoma should be reported to the referring physician. A large fibroid reported in the cervical region will alert the obstetrician to potential difficulties during labor and delivery. A degenerating fibroid in close proximity to the placental implantation site may be a potential threat to the continuing pregnancy. Such findings are easily identified during ultrasound examination. A pedunculated uterine fibroid positioned posterior to the uterus can suggest uterine size greater than expected dates, as it displaces the uterus anterior and cephalad. A pedunculated fibroid may be separate from the uterus and mistaken for a solid ovarian mass. This dilemma is discussed in greater detail in the section on gynecologic ultrasound.

Less common causes of uterine masses are uterine carcinoma and duplication. Uterine carcinoma has an ultrasound appearance similar to a degenerating fibroid. The texture of the mass often is uneven and mixed. If hemorrhage is present, through transmission will be identified. Cases of uterine duplication result in size-dates discrepancy early in pregnancy. The gravid uterus is easily recognized, but the nongravid uterus may be confused for an ovarian lesion. The diagnosis is made by lining up the gravid uterus with the vagina and demonstrating continuity of the two on longitudinal oblique scans. Decidual reaction often is present in the nongravid uterus, suggesting the diagnosis. Aligning the nongravid uterus with the vagina also demonstrates continuity.

Large ovarian masses may elevate the uterus out of the pelvis, causing the obstetrician to assume a fundal height larger than expected from the patient's menstrual history. If the mass is situated cephalad to the fundus, the top of the mass may be misinterpreted as the fundus of the uterus and lead to a falsely large fundal height.

Simple ovarian cysts are echo-free masses with sharp borders and enhanced through transmission. Multiloculated cysts are fluid-filled masses with various curvilinear echoes present inside. Dermoids have a varying ultrasonic appearance, depending on their contents. Ovarian tumors have echoes throughout, indicating their solid nature. Any of these ovarian masses may be present in conjunction with pregnancy. Ultrasound will locate the mass, estimate its size, and evaluate its texture. This information often leads to the correct diagnosis of the nature of the mass and assists the obstetrician in determining whether surgical intervention is necessary.

There are other masses in the pelvis that can elevate the uterus and lead to a size-dates discrepancy. These include hydrosalpinx, tubo-ovarian abscesses, endometriosis, ectopic pelvis kidney, stool in the rectosigmoid, and bowel masses. These entities have varying ultrasonographic appearances, which are discussed later in this volume.

Incompetent Cervix

Incompetent cervix presents in the second trimester as a painless, bloodless abortion with minimal warning. It is frequently secondary to previous trauma such as a difficult delivery or previous D and C. Other etiologies such as emotional factors or a weakness of the cervical muscle ring have been entertained.

Ultrasound examination of the lower uterine segment and endocervical canal now can confirm the clinical impression of an incompetent cervix. Most often, these patients present with two or three previous abortions in the second trimester. If such a patient is encountered, an ultrasound examination of the endocervical canal should be undertaken.

The technique for examination of the endocervical canal is extremely important. Transverse scans should initially be obtained perpendicular to the long axis of the cervix. The right and left borders of the cervix should be marked on the patient's skin. The transducer arm should then be realigned parallel to the long axis of the cervix for the longitudinal scans. Often, this is a midline scan; occasionally, however, the cervix is oriented obliquely to the right or left. The initial transverse scans will delineate the oblique angle of the cervix. The longitudinal scan should then begin to the right or the left and proceed at half-centimeter intervals through the entire cervix. The majority of the scans will demonstrate the echogenic muscle of the cervix, but when the midportion of the cervix is approached, a strong linear echo arising from the endocervical canal will be noted within the muscle tissues of the cervix. This strong linear echo should be visualized in its entirety, from the external to the internal os. If an incompetent cervix is present, sonolucency due to amniotic fluid will be noted in the endocervical canal. This may extend nearly the entire length of the endocervical canal. It is extremely important that adequate bladder distension be present to ensure adequate visualization of the lower uterine segment and cervix. It should also be noted that overdistention of the urinary bladder can lead to collapse of the cervix from the increased pressure in the urinary bladder. Therefore, if on initial examination the urinary bladder appears overly distended, the patient should partially void and then be reexamined to determine if the lower uterine segment distends and fluid is noted in the endocervical canal (Sarti, Sample, Hobel, and Staisch 1979).

It is extremely difficult and unusual to visualize an incompetent cervix with ultrasound prior to the fourteenth or fifteenth week. At this early stage of pregnancy, the volume of the fluid and fetus within the uterus is not adequate to cause distention of the lower uterine segment and cervix. By the seventeenth or eighteenth week of pregnancy, however, an incompetent cervix can be visualized with ultrasound.

In any patient clinically suspected of having an incompetent cervix, an ultrasound examination of the lower uterine area should be performed serially at 2- or 3-week intervals until about the twenty-fourth week. By this stage of pregnancy, if fluid is not identified in the endocervical canal by ultrasound, it is extremely unlikely an incompetent cervix is present.

Ectopic Pregnancy

The diagnosis of an ectopic pregnancy is often difficult and frustrating. The clinical symptoms of spotting and pelvic pain in a woman who has recently missed her last period can represent various entities ranging from innocuous to potentially fatal. These mild symptoms may be the initial signs of an ectopic pregnancy with its grave consequences. In this clinical setting, ultrasound plays a helpful role in the decision-making process of the obstetrician. It is important that the information obtained from an ultrasound examination be placed in proper prospective. Ultrasound may provide critical information to the referring obstetrician, but it does have certain limitations. Its major purpose in this situation is to confirm an intrauterine pregnancy.

In order to understand the role and limitations of ultrasound in the workup of a patient suspected of having an ectopic pregnancy, it is necessary to review the ultrasonic findings in normal early pregnancy. As discussed earlier in this section, a gestational sac is first visualized at 5 to 6 menstrual weeks. The embryo is not visible until the seventh menstrual week. The ultrasonic diagnosis of an intrauterine pregnancy cannot be made with 100% certainty until an embryo is visualized in the uterine cavity. If an embryo is identified in the uterine cavity, an ectopic pregnancy is ruled out.

Unfortunately, many patients suspected of having an ectopic pregnancy develop symptoms prior to 7 menstrual weeks, before an embryo can be identified by ultrasound. At this stage in a normal pregnancy only a gestational sac is visualized. A false sac, or pseudosac, of an ectopic pregnancy may be present and mistaken for a normal intrauterine pregnancy (Marks, Filly, Callen, and Laing 1979). This false sac occurs secondary to highly reflective decidua surrounding an echo-free area of hemorrhage and can be very similar in appearance to a normal 5- to 6-week sac. Therefore, visualization of a 1- to 2-cm sac in the uterus does not definitely confirm an intrauterine pregnancy. Very often there are clues, such as the thickness of the surrounding echoes or visualization of the yolk sac, that may suggest an intrauterine pregnancy. Nevertheless, visualization of the embryo within the uterus is necessary to rule out an ectopic pregnancy.

Another diagnostic problem is that ectopic pregnancies are varied in appearance. The classic ultrasound picture of a well-circumscribed gestational sac containing an embryo situated outside the uterus in the adnexal region is an uncommon occurrence. Since hormonal stimulation supports the developing decidua, the uterine cavity often will have strong central echoes or even develop a false sac. The remainder of the pelvis may contain a cystic mass, gestational sac, fetal structures, fluid in the cul-de-sac, or any combination of these (Kobayashi, Hellman, and Cromb 1972; Rogers, Shaub, and Wilson 1977). In very early ectopic pregnancies that are too small to be seen, ultrasound of the pelvis may be completely negative with no masses or fluid identified and an empty uterus.

With all of these drawbacks, what is the role of diagnostic ultrasound in the workup of a patient suspected of having an ectopic pregnancy? The primary function of the ultrasonographer is to inform the obstetrician if an intrauterine pregnancy is present. Ectopic pregnancy is ruled out in the presence of this diagnosis. Another important diagnosis is impending abortion. This not only rules out ectopic pregnancy, but it also warns the obstetrician about continued viability. An ectopic pregnancy can be definitely diagnosed when the embryo is seen outside the uterus. Finally, there are times when neither intrauterine nor ectopic pregnancy may be visualized by ultrasound. This is a common finding and warrants close clinical observation since ectopic pregnancy has not been ruled out.

Fetal Death

An ultrasound examination often is ordered when there is a question of fetal viability. The patient may not feel any activity for several days or the obstetrician may be unable to detect fetal cardiac activity. By the seventh menstrual or fifth conceptual week fetal cardiac activity is easily visualized with real-time ultrasound. At this time, the crown–rump length is about 1 cm. Numerous ultrasonic signs are suggestive of fetal demise, but failure to visualize fetal cardiac activity is the only sign diagnostic of fetal demise. Since the fetal outline is easily localized with ultrasound, the fetal cardiac examination concentrates in the region of the fetal thorax. Close scrutiny of this area with real time and Doppler easily detects fetal cardiac activity. If nothing is detected, a systematic approach of scanning the fetus from head to pelvis numerous times will confirm the absence of cardiac activity.

On static ultrasound images, there are various signs suggesting fetal demise that necessitate a real-time examination for confirmation. There may be a coarsening of the fetal outline involving the fetal head, fetal body, or both (Gottesfeld 1970; Leopold and Asher 1975; Sanders and Conrad 1975). This is secondary to edema, which may become so severe that a double outline is visualized surrounding the fetus. Following demise, degeneration of tissue occurs, leading to deformity of fetal echoes. Overlapping of fetal skull, severe angulation of the fetal spine, distortion of intracranial echoes, and poor anatomic detail in the fetal thorax and abdomen are all signs of degeneration or necrosis. When any of these signs are visualized, real-time examination of the fetal thorax is indicated to determine whether fetal cardiac activity is present.

Fetal Anatomy and Abnormalities

Continuous improvement in the resolution of ultrasound equipment has resulted in better image quality, so that ultrasound examination of the fetus recently has taken on a new role. Years ago, obstetricians were satisfied to know that a fetus was lying in a certain position and was alive. Today, the fetus is treated as a patient and undergoes a physical examination in which diagnostic ultrasound replaces the palpating hand and observing eye, yielding information that is truly remarkable in its detail.

Intracranial detail such as the falx, third ventricle, and other midline structures are visualized. The lateral ventricles and midbrain are seen routinely. The cerebellum, orbits, base of skull, nose, and mouth are identified when the fetus is in correct position. Evaluation of the fetal thorax, heart, and lungs is also possible by ultrasound (Garrett, Kossoff, and Lawrence 1975; Kossoff, Garrett, and Radavonovich 1974). The cardiac chambers, interventricular septum, and mitral and tricuspid valves are seen with real-time scanners. The anatomy of the abdomen, including liver, umbilical vein, kidneys, gallbladder, urinary bladder, stomach, and bowel loops have characteristic ultrasound appearances (Flanigan and Butiny 1977; Lee and Blake 1977). Changes in the size of the stomach, bowel loops, and urinary bladder can be recorded during or between examinations. Fetal activity such as breathing, extremity movement, and urinary bladder emptying can be documented. The size and shape of osseous structures, including the extremities, clavicles, and scapulae are subject to scrutiny. Ultrasonic evaluation of the fetal spine often is critically important in a workup for fetal well-being. Examination of the fetal spine is quite difficult and requires a great deal of experience. The cervical, thoracic, lumbar, and sacral spine are visualized in transverse and longitudinal planes. Adequate visualization of various areas of the fetal spine are dependent on fetal position, and complete examination may necessitate several studies in order to change fetal orientation.

All of these normal anatomic structures are visible at present with ultrasound. A normal fetal physical examination is a common occurrence since the great majority of pregnancies are healthy and uneventful episodes. Nevertheless, more and more fetal examinations are turning up questionable or abnormal anatomic findings as equipment improves and as the level of experience of the ultrasonographer increases. Correct anatomic interpretations require an accurate three-dimensional concept of fetal position during scanning. This concept may change continually during an examination as the fetus moves. Once the ultrasonographer loses orientation, interpretative errors increase. Therefore, the ultrasonographer continually is reevaluating fetal position and adjusting the scanner according to fetal lie. This increases the diagnostic accuracy of detecting fetal abnormalities.

For obstetricians entering the field of ultrasonography, detection of fetal abnormalities is the area of greatest uncertainty. Most novice ultrasonographers will be misguided by the expectation that most pregnancies will result in a normal baby and may thus dismiss unusual or unfamiliar fetal ultrasound findings. Such inexperience may be responsible for a current increase in malpractice suits stemming from missed diagnoses of fetal abnormalities during ultrasonic evaluation of the pregnancy. Regrettably, the future of fetal ultrasound is clouded by these unresolved medicolegal difficulties.

Abnormalities of the fetal head usually are identified when the examiner is attempting to measure the biparietal diameter. Anencephaly presents as a cluster of echoes in the area of the fetal head, and a typical measurement of biparietal diameter cannot be obtained. Since a biparietal diameter is visible in 100% of patients by the fifteenth menstrual week, anencephaly is diagnosed easily at this time. Microcephaly is more difficult to diagnose, especially early in pregnancy. It is more dependent upon recognition of a disproportion between the fetal head and body or extremity. Serial exams often are necessary to document a normal growth rate to the fetal abdomen or limb and an abnormally slow growth rate to the fetal head.

Hydrocephalus can be diagnosed by noting increased growth rate of the biparietal diameter or a disproportionately large head in relation to body size (Freeman et al. 1977). A biparietal diameter greater than 10.7 cm is considered consistent with hydrocephalus (Sanders and Conrad 1975). Babies of diabetic mothers can be quite large at term, however, and care must be taken in diagnosing hydrocephalus solely on the basis of head size. Visualization of dilated lateral ventricles confirms the diagnosis. It is important to remember that there is a normal variation of the relative size of the lateral ventricles compared to cerebrum. From 14 to approximately 20 or 22 weeks the ventricles are quite prominent; by 26 to 28 weeks they approach a more normal ratio compared to cerebrum. Hydrocephalus often is wrongly diagnosed from 15 to 22 weeks because of lack of appreciation of this normal variation. If hydrocephalus is suspected at 15 weeks, serial studies at 2- to 3-week intervals are suggested. If hydrocephalus is present, the ventricular ratio will more often increase over time. The choroid plexus also helps in diagnosing hydrocephalus. It is a highly echogenic structure within the posterior aspect of the lateral ventricles. In hydrocephalus the choroid plexus usually has a smaller, more shrunken appearance than normal. Another common difficulty in evaluating hydrocephalus is that often only one lateral ventricle is visualized as dilated. The dilated ventricle is always the deep or far ventricle. The near ventricle does not usually appear to be dilated. This feature, however, is secondary to reverberation artifacts arising from the near fetal skull. The reverberation echoes are displayed in the near dilated ventricle, masking its true appearance. Cautious scanning, repositioning the fetus, and experience in scanning help in recognizing this problem.

As noted, evaluation of the fetal spine is quite difficult. Since an elevated alpha-fetoprotein often is associated with a neural tube defect, close examination of the fetal spine is necessary in the presence of such a laboratory finding. Distortion of the fetal spine echoes or a mass may be evident. In the case of a meningocele or meningomyelocele a mass in close proximity to the fetal spine is seen if the mass is large enough. Very often these appear as cystic or multicystic structures. A cystic hygroma in the posterior neck region will have an ultrasonic appearance very similar to that of a meningocele. In these instances, close examination of the cervical spine for abnormalities helps to differentiate the two entities.

Abnormalities of the fetal abdomen often are secondary to obstruction of the gastrointestinal or genitourinary systems. When a gastrointestinal obstruction is present, polyhydramnios often is found in association with the pregnancy. Fluid-filled structures such as the stomach, bowel loops, and urinary bladder are seen routinely in the normal fetus. Dilated, obstructed bowel appears distended and remains unchanged between examinations. These findings in conjunction with polyhydramnios lead to the diagnosis of gastrointestinal obstruction. Such entities as esophageal, duodenal, or jejunal atresia can be diagnosed by ultrasound studies.

Abnormalities of the genitourinary system often are accompanied by oligohydramnios. Fluid in the renal areas may be secondary to hydronephrosis or multicystic kidney. If the fetal abdomen is enlarged and bilateral renal obstruction is present, prune-belly syndrome is a likely possibility. Other abdominal abnormalities include omphalocele, ascites, mesenteric cysts, and ovarian cysts. Evaluation of patients at high risk for dwarfism is also possible since the proximal and distal extremities can be accurately measured.

References

Brown, R. E. *Ultrasonography. Basic principles and clinical applications.* St. Louis: Warren H. Green, Inc., 1975.

Campbell, S. The prediction of fetal maturity by ultrasonic measurement of the biparietal diameter. *Br. J. Obstet. Gynaecol.* 76:603, 1969.

Campbell, S., and Dewhurst, C. J. Quintuplet pregnancy diagnosed and assessed by ultrasonic compound scanning. *Lancet* 1:101, 1970.

Donald, I. Sonar as a method of studying prenatal development. *J. Pediatr.* 75:326, 1969.

Donald, I., and Brown, T. G. Demonstration of tissue interfaces within the body by ultrasonic echo sounding. *Brit. J. Radiol.* 34:539, 1961.

Donald, I.; MacVicar, J.; and Brown, T. G. Investigation of abdominal masses by pulsed ultrasound. *Lancet* 1:1188, 1958.

Donald, I.; Morley, P.; and Barnett, E. The diagnosis of blighted ovum by sonar. *Br. J. Obstet. Gynaecol.* 79:304, 1972.

Flamme, P. Ultrasonic fetal cephalometry: percentile curve. *Br. Med. J.* 3:384, 1972.

Flanigan, D. J., and Butiny, J. H. Ultrasonic imaging of normal intrauterine anatomy. *J. Clin. Ultrasound* 5:334, 1977.

Freeman, R. T. et al. The diagnosis of fetal hydrocephalus before viability. *Obstet. Gynecol.* 49:109, 1977.

Garrett, W. J.; Grunwald, G.; and Robinson, D. E. Prenatal diagnosis of fetal polycystic kidney by ultrasound. *Aust. N. Z. J. Obstet. Gynaecol.* 10:7, 1970.

Garrett, W. J.; Kossoff, G.; and Lawrence, R. Grey scale echography in the diagnosis of hydrops due to fetal lung tumors. *J. Clin. Ultrasound* 3:45, 1975.

Ghorashi, B., and Gottesfeld, K. R. The grey scale appearance of the normal pregnancy from 14 to 16 weeks of gestation. *J. Clin. Ultrasound* 15:195, 1977.

Gottesfeld, K. R. The ultrasonic diagnosis of intrauterine fetal death. *Am. J. Obstet. Gynecol.* 108:623, 1970.

Gottesfeld, K. R. Ultrasound in obstetrics & gynecology. *Semin. Roentgenol.* 10:305, 1975.

Gottesfeld, K. R.; Thompson, H. E.; Holmes, J. H.; and Taylor, E. S. Ultrasonic placentography—a new method for placental localization. *Am. J. Obstet. Gynecol.* 96:538, 1966.

Hellman, L. M. et al. Growth and development of the human fetus prior to the twentieth week of gestation. *Am. J. Obstet. Gynecol.* 103:789, 1969.

Hellman, L. M.; Kobayashi, M.; and Cromb, E. Ultrasonic diagnosis of embryonic malformations. *Am. J. Obstet. Gynecol.* 115:615, 1973.

Horger, E. D.; Kreutner, A. K.; Underwood, P. B. Ultrasonic diagnosis of low implantation preceding placenta previa. *Am. J. Obstet. Gynecol.* 120:1119, 1974.

King, D. L. Placental ultrasonography. *J. Clin. Ultrasound* 1:21, 1973.

Kobayashi, M.; Hellman, L. M.; and Cromb, E. *Atlas of ultrasonography in obstetrics and gynecology.* New York: Appleton-Century-Crofts, 1972.

Kohorn, E. I., and Kaufman, M. Sonar in the first trimester of pregnancy. *Obstet. Gynecol.* 44:473, 1974.

Kossoff, G.; Garrett, W. J.; and Radavonovich, G. Grey scale echography in obstetrics and gynecology. *Australas. Radiol.* 18:62, 1974.

Langman, J. *Medical embryology.* Baltimore: The Williams & Wilkins Co., 1969.

Lee, T. G., and Blake, S. Prenatal fetal abdominal ultrasonography and diagnosis. *Radiology* 124:475, 1977.

Leopold, G. R. Diagnostic ultrasound in the detection of molar pregnancy. *Radiology* 98:171, 1971.

Leopold, G. R., and Asher, W. M. *Fundamentals of abdominal and pelvic ultrasonography.* Philadelphia: W. B. Saunders Co., 1975.

Levi, S. The use of ultrasonic biparietal diameter measurement of the fetus in assessing gestational age. *Acta Obstet. Gynecol. Scand.* 50:179, 1971.

Levi, S. Ultrasonic assessment of the high rate of human multiple pregnancy in the first trimester. *J. Clin. Ultrasound* 4:3, 1976.

Marks, W. M.; Filly, R. A.; Callen, P. W.; and Laing, F. C. The decidual cast of ectopic pregnancy: a confusing ultrasonographic appearance. *Radiology* 133:451, 1979.

Robinson, H. P. Detection of fetal heart movement in first trimester of pregnancy using pulsed ultrasound. *Br. Med. J.* 4:466, 1972.

Robinson, H. P., and Caines, J. S. Sonar evidence of early pregnancy failure in patients with twin conceptions. *Br. J. Obstet. Gynaecol.* 84:22, 1977.

Rogers, W. F.; Shaub, M. S.; and Wilson, R. Chronic ectopic pregnancy: ultrasonic diagnosis. *J. Clin. Ultrasound* 5:257, 1977.

Sanders, R. C., and Conrad, M. R. Sonography in obstetrics. *Radiol. Clin. North Am.* 13:435, 1975.

Sarti, D. A.; Sample, W. F.; Hobel, C. J.; and Staisch, K. J. Ultrasonic visualization of a dilated cervix during pregnancy. *Radiology* 130:417, 1979.

Scheer, K. Ultrasound in twin gestation. *J. Clin. Ultrasound* 2:197, 1974.

Thompson, H. E. Ultrasonic diagnostic procedures in obstetrics and gynecology. *J. Clin. Ultrasound* 1:160, 1973.

Winsberg, F. Echographic changes with placental aging. *J. Clin. Ultrasound* 1:52, 1973.

CASES
Normal Gestational Sac   I.

Fertilization takes place in the distal third of the fallopian tubes, approximately 2 weeks after menstruation. The fertilized ovum travels down the fallopian tube and reaches the uterus approximately 2–3 days after fertilization. The blastocyst then floats in the uterine cavity and finally embeds in the uterine mucosa after about 3 or 4 more days. Therefore, approximately 7 days after fertilization, the blastocyst has finally embedded itself within the uterine mucosa. The blastocyst cannot be visualized at this time because of its small size. At about two weeks after fertilization, however, ultrasound can visualize the first evidence of a beginning gestational sac.

Figure 1 is a longitudinal scan of the uterus with a strong central echo in the fundal region; this is the beginning gestational sac. This is approximately 2–2½ weeks after fertilization, which would correspond to 4–4½ weeks after the last menstruation. This is the earliest visualization of the gestational sac. We do not see any central fluid at this time. The gestational sac continues to enlarge. In figure 2 the gestational sac is seen at approximately 5 menstrual weeks. A central sonolucency within the gestational sac represents the amniotic fluid. This is a more typical appearance of the gestational sac with the strong surrounding echoes of the chorionic villi and the decidual reaction. The surrounding echoes are very important, for they give an impression of the normal vascularity to the gestational sac. The high-amplitude echoes are a good sign of prominent chorionic villi developing within the uterus.

Figure 3 is another longitudinal scan at approximately 5–6 menstrual weeks. Again, the strong surrounding echoes of the chorionic villi are seen. The central portion of the gestational sac is fluid-filled. The embryo is not visualized at this time, since it is too

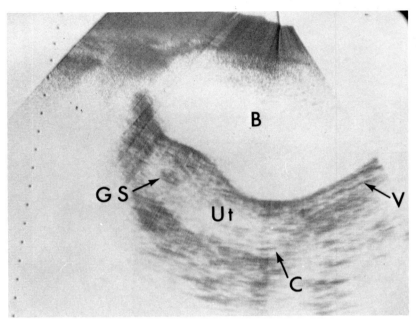

Fig. 1

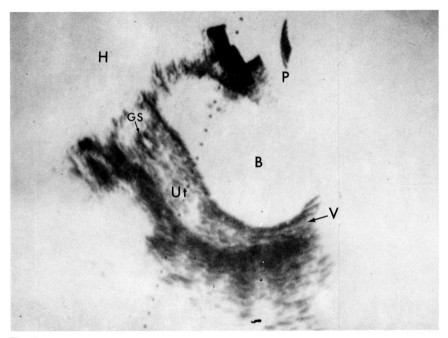

Fig. 2

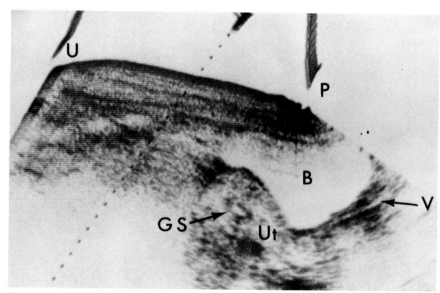

Fig. 3

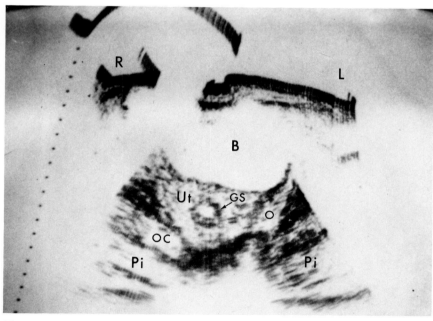

Fig. 4

small to be detected with ultrasound. The important finding is the strong surrounding echoes of the gestational sac, which indicate a normal adequate blood supply.

Figure 4 is a transverse scan of the pregnant uterus at approximately 6 menstrual weeks. Again we see the strong surrounding echoes of the chorionic villi in the gestational sac. Fluid is noted centrally without evidence of an embryo at this time. An ovarian cyst is on the right side, consistent with a corpus luteum cyst of pregnancy.

B	=	Urinary bladder
C	=	Cervix
GS	=	Gestational sac
H	=	Head
L	=	Left
O	=	Ovary
OC	=	Ovarian cyst
P	=	Level of the symphysis pubis
Pi	=	Piriformis muscles
R	=	Right
U	=	Umbilical level
Ut	=	Uterus
V	=	Vagina

Normal Gestational Sac   II.

The gestational sac continues to grow in size during the first 10 weeks. It grows at approximately 1 cm per week in mean diameter. Therefore, normal growth is easy to measure in serial examinations. The embryo can be seen at approximately the seventh menstrual week, when it attains a size large enough for ultrasonic detection. Figure 5 is a longitudinal scan in which we see a gestational sac situated in the fundus of the uterus. It is approximately 2–3 cm in diameter. Strong surrounding echoes indicate good vascular supply to the chorionic villi. A small echo (arrow) is noted in the central portion of the gestational sac. This is the early detection of the embryo by ultrasound. The embryo is approximately 5 mm in size by the seventh menstrual week.

Figure 6 is a longitudinal scan of the pregnant uterus at approximately 8 weeks gestation. The fetus has enlarged to approximately 1 cm in diameter. It is easily recognizable within the amniotic fluid of the gestational sac. The gestational sac is now strongly surrounded by echoes that are thicker on one side. The thicker portion of the gestational sac will become the placenta, while the thinner portion will eventually atrophy and completely disappear. That portion of the gestational sac that is away from the implantation site eventually outgrows its blood supply and atrophies completely. This leads to the disappearance of the gestational sac.

Occasionally, two fluid-filled areas are seen within the uterus separated by a curvilinear septum (figs. 7 and 8). This is an indication of a twin pregnancy. In figure 7, we see two fluid-filled sacs separated by a curvilinear septum. In one sac the internal echoes indicate a fetus. The other sac is completely clear. This could represent an anembryonic pregnancy on one side. Close examination of the gestational sac, however, is necessary, since we may not be passing the transducer beam over the site of the fetus. Figure 8 is the same patient. A fetus is visualized in both sides of the gestational sac. This is a

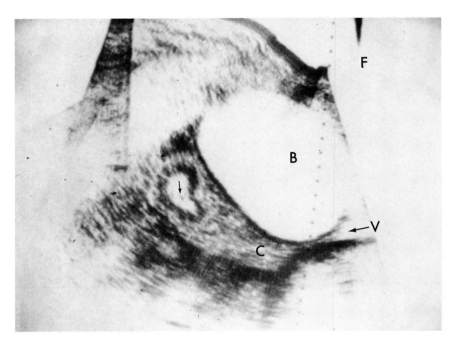

Fig. 5

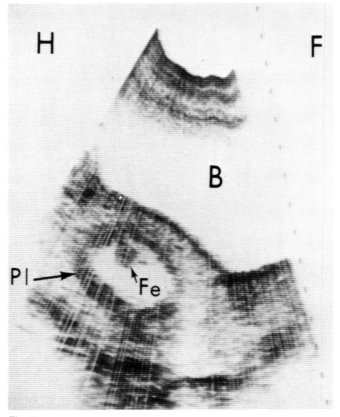

Fig. 6

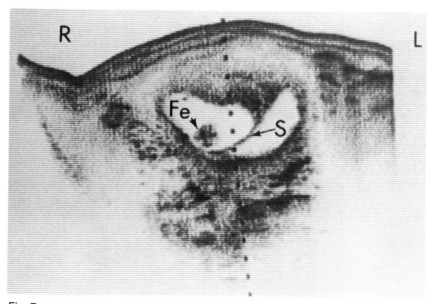

Fig. 7

normal twin pregnancy with separate amniotic cavities.

Arrows	=	Early embryo
B	=	Urinary bladder
C	=	Cervix
F	=	Foot
Fe	=	Fetus
H	=	Head
L	=	Left
Pl	=	Placenta
R	=	Right
S	=	Septum separating a twin pregnancy
V	=	Vagina

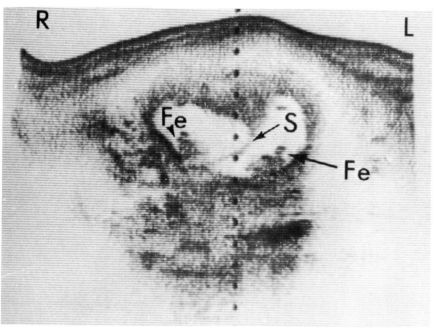

Fig. 8

Normal Gestational Sac   III.

As the gestational sac continues to enlarge, the region of the placenta becomes thicker. The area that will no longer be the placenta continues to thin out and eventually disappears. Figure 9 is a longitudinal scan of the gestational sac is approximately 9 weeks' gestation. Here we see a thickened placenta situated posteriorly. The anterior portion of the gestational sac is less echogenic and much thinner; this indicates normal atrophy. The myometrium situated posterior to the placenta has a lighter echo pattern to it than the highly echogenic placenta. A corpus luteum cyst is seen in the region of the cul-de-sac.

Figure 10 is a longitudinal scan at approximately 9–10 weeks' gestation. Again we see a thickened echogenic region posteriorly; this represents the placental site. Thinning and decreasing echogenicity to the surrounding gestational sac, secondary to normal vascular atrophy, is seen in the anterior portion (arrows).

Figure 11 is a transverse scan with a thick posterior placenta. Again, the anterior portion of the gestational sac is much thinner. This normal disappearance of vascular supply is very important to appreciate. It can become very difficult to diagnose an impending abortion around 10 weeks of pregnancy because of the normal atrophic appearance to the gestational sac. If decreased echogenicity is seen at 6, 7, or 8 weeks, the diagnosis of an impending abortion is more likely.

Figure 12 is a pregnancy at approximately 11 weeks. This is a time in which the gestational sac has disappeared. The placenta is situated posteriorly. It is quite thick and has a high echogenicity which indicates good vascular supply. It is important, however, to notice the surrounding portion of the gestational sac. We no longer see the thick surrounding echoes (arrows). Instead, amniotic fluid in contact with myometrial echoes is visualized. It is around the eleventh to twelfth week that the gestional sac disappears, and only placental tissue is evident.

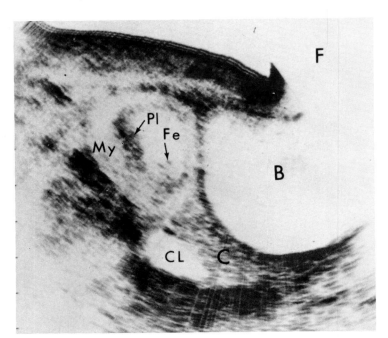

Fig. 9

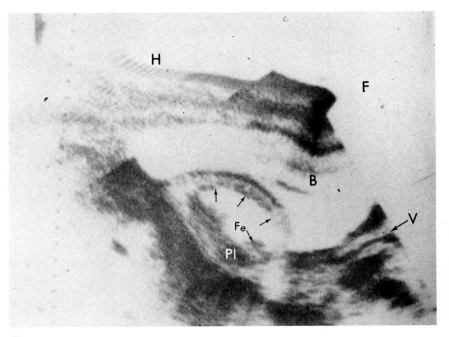

Fig. 10

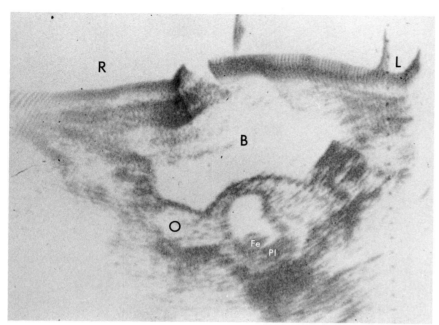

Fig. 11

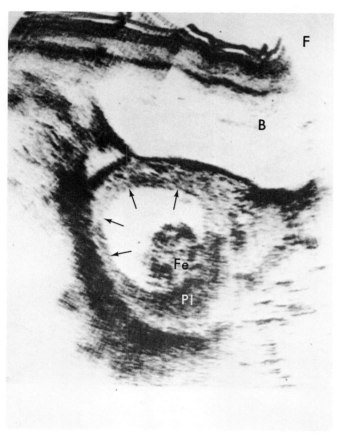

Fig. 12

Arrows = thinning vascular supply to the gestational sac (fig. 10)
Arrows = Eventual disappearance of the gestational sac (fig. 12)
B = Urinary bladder
C = Cervix
CL = Corpus luteum cyst
F = Foot
Fe = Fetus
H = Head
L = Left
My = Myometrium
O = Right Ovary
Pl = Placenta
R = Right
V = Vagina

Abnormal Gestational Sac   I.

Numerous ultrasonic signs can indicate an abnormal gestational sac. In figure 13 a longitudinal scan demonstrates a gestational sac without the usual round or oval appearance. In the caudal portion of the gestational sac we see a pointed segment. A pointed segment is a strong indication that an abnormal sac is present. The same patient was scanned in the transverse plane (fig. 14). Here we see an uneven thickness and echogenicity to the surrounding echoes of the gestational sac. Areas of thinner echogenicity (arrows) present on the anterior and posterior segments of the gestational sac (fig. 14). This is compatible with decreased vascular supply to an abnormal sac. The vascularity of a gestational sac can be visualized by the thickness and strength of the surrounding echoes. Here we have evidence of an abnormal vascular supply.

The patient was brought back 10 days later (figs. 15 and 16). Figure 15 is a longitudinal scan indicating marked decrease in the surrounding echoes (arrows). A transverse scan confirms the decreased echogenicity. Also of extreme importance is the fact that the gestational sac did not increase in size. If there is any question as to an abnormal sac, the patient should be studied 7–10 days later. In this time period, the mean diameter of the sac should increase at least 1 cm. The main findings of this case are the pointed segment and decreased echogenicity indicating an abnormal gestational sac.

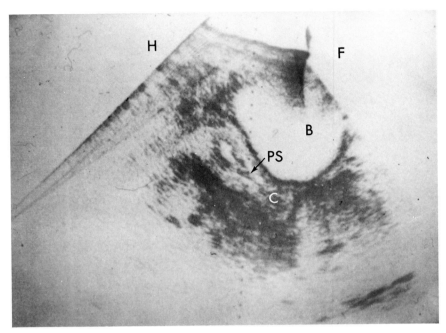

Fig. 13

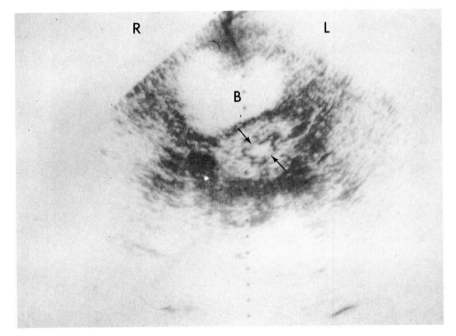

Fig. 14

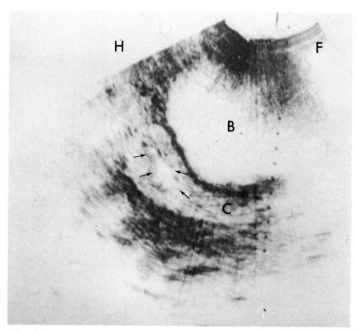

Fig. 15

Arrows = Decreased vascular supply to the gestational sac
B = Urinary bladder
C = Cervix
F = Foot
H = Head
L = Left
PS = Pointed segment
R = Right

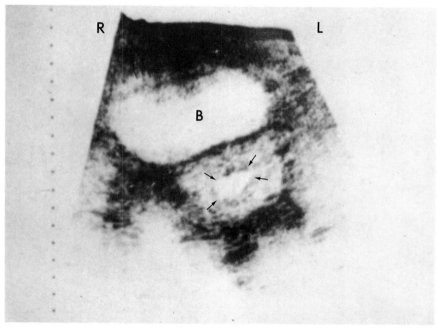

Fig. 16

Abnormal Gestational Sac   II.

Figure 17 is an example of an abnormal gestational sac with evidence not only of a pointed segment but also an actual break in the gestational sac. The caudal portion of the gestational sac is markedly abnormal compared with the previous normals.

Often, a double gestational sac is present. This may represent a normal twin gestation, but the possibility of an abnormal pregnancy should also be considered. Figure 18 is a longitudinal scan with two gestational sacs (numbers 1 and 2) in the mid portion of the uterus. It is important to notice that a small fluid collection is present above the two gestational sacs. This patient went on to have a complete abortion approximately 1 week later.

The implantation site of a normal gestational sac is usually fundal or mid-uterine in location. Occasionally, a low implantation site is seen (fig. 19). The gestational sac is located in the cervical region of the uterus. The patient was examined 1 week later, and a complete abortion occurred (fig. 20). Here we see no evidence of the gestational sac. Low implantation may indicate an impending abortion. These cases should be followed carefully.

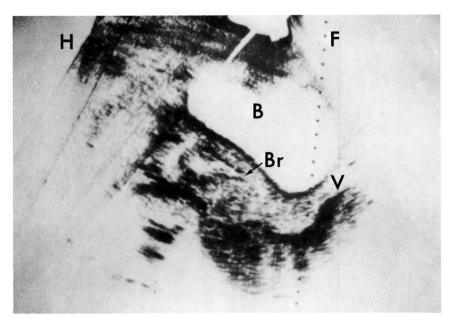

Fig. 17

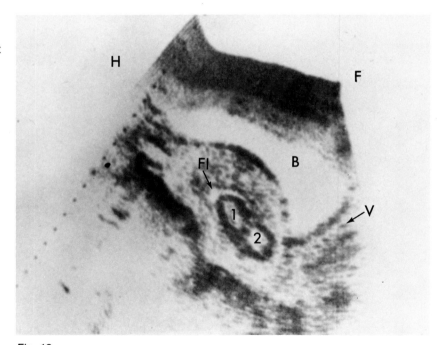

Fig. 18

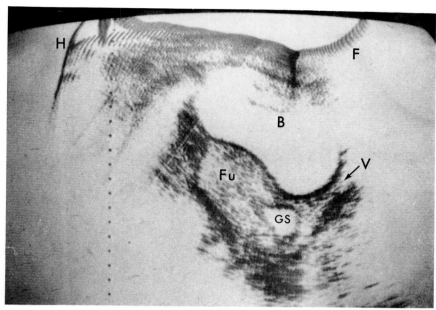

B	= Urinary bladder
Br	= Break in the gestational sac
C	= Cervix
F	= Foot
Fl	= Fluid above the gestational sac
Fu	= Fundus of the uterus
GS	= Low-lying gestational sac
H	= Head
Numbers 1 and 2	= Two gestational sacs
P	= Symphysis pubis
V	= Vagina

Fig. 19

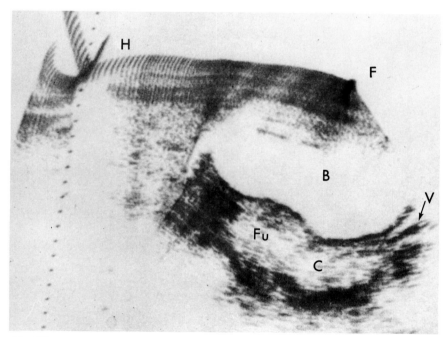

Fig. 20

Abnormal Gestational Sac III.

Frequently a large amount of fluid is seen in the gestational sac, but without evidence of any fetal echoes. This has been termed an anembryonic pregnancy or a blighted ovum. A longitudinal scan of the uterus (fig. 21) demonstrates a large amount of fluid in the gestational sac. The surrounding echoes however, are quite thin and weak, indicating an abnormal pregnancy. A break in the gestational sac with some fragmentation of the surrounding echoes supports this. Figure 22 is a transverse scan of an anembryonic pregnancy with markedly weak surrounding echoes (arrows). This indicates a poor vascular supply to the gestational sac. We do not find evidence of any fetal echoes within this rather large gestational sac. Once a gestational sac reaches a size of approximately 2–3 cm, it should demonstrate fetal echoes. If fetal echoes are not present on a close and meticulous examination, then an anembryonic pregnancy can be diagnosed.

Figures 23 and 24 are longitudinal and transverse scans of a patient with an anembryonic pregnancy. Here we see an empty gestational sac. Weak, thin surrounding echoes (arrows) indicate poor vascular supply to this pregnancy. When there is no evidence of a placental site with a gestational sac of this size, an anembryonic pregnancy can be diagnosed. This gestational sac is approximately 7–8 cm. By this time a markedly thick portion which will eventually be the placental site is seen. The fetus should also be quite large by this time.

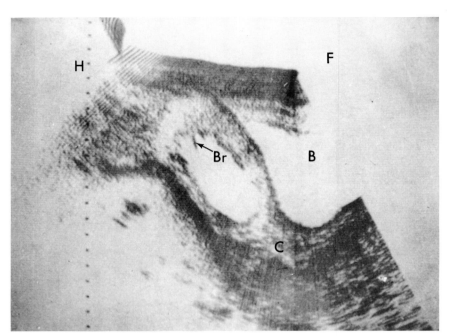

Fig. 21

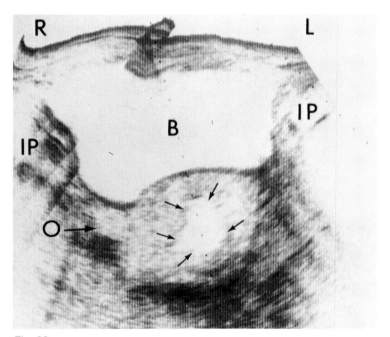

Fig. 22

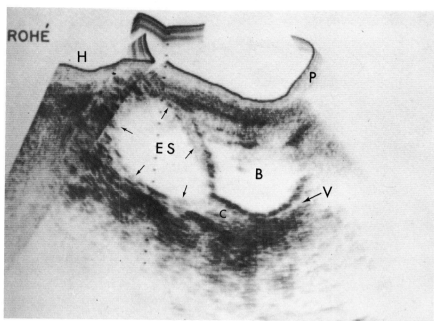

Fig. 23

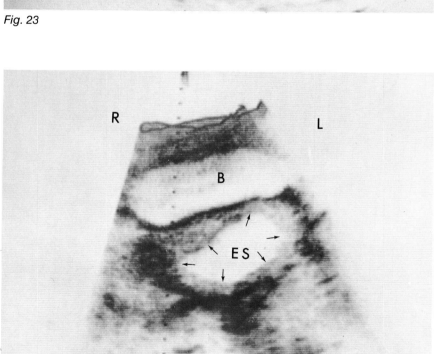

Fig. 24

Arrows	=	Weak and thin surrounding echoes indicating an abnormal gestational sac
B	=	Urinary bladder
Br	=	Break in the gestational sac indicating fragmentation
C	=	Cervix
ES	=	Empty gestational sac
F	=	Foot
H	=	Head
IP	=	Iliopsoas muscle
L	=	Left
O	=	Right Ovary
R	=	Right

Incomplete Abortion   I.

Often, a patient is sent for an ultrasound examination to determine whether or not she has aborted completely. Clinically, she will be having some spotting and pain. It is not felt that the pregnancy is viable, but it must be determined whether or not the uterus has completely emptied itself.

Figures 25 and 26 are typical of a patient who has had an incomplete abortion. Strong echoes (arrows) are seen in the endometrial cavity which is somewhat thicker than we usually see with normal menstruation. In the right clinical setting, however, the findings are compatible with an incomplete abortion. The patient can be followed for several weeks to see whether or not the uterus empties itself completely. If central echoes are still present over a prolonged period of time, a D and C should be performed.

Figures 27 and 28 are of an incomplete abortion which has gone on for longer than 3 years. The patient had an abortion 3 years previously without complete emptying of the uterus. Strong central echoes (arrows) are seen within the mid portion of the uterus. In this instance, shadowing is distal to the echoes indicating calcification within the mid portion of the uterus. The retained products of conception actually contained bony structures from the fetus.

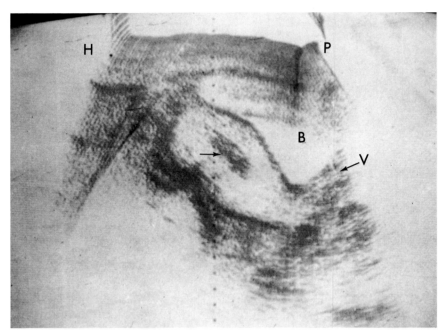

Fig. 25

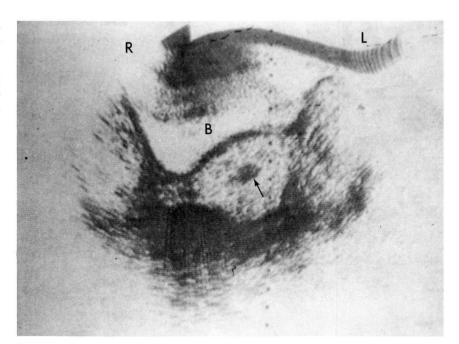

Fig. 26

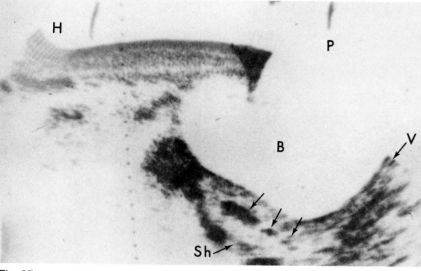

Fig. 27

Arrows = Strong central echoes indicating an incomplete abortion
B = Urinary bladder
FT = Left fallopian tube
H = Head
L = Left
P = Level of the symphysis pubis
R = Right
Sh = Shadowing behind retained fetal products
V = Vagina

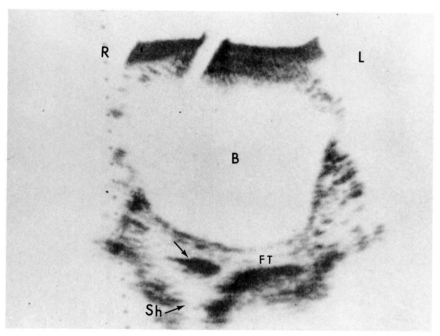

Fig. 28

Incomplete Abortion   II.

Figure 29 is another example of re-tained products (arrows) within the central portion of the uterus. It almost appears to be an incomplete sac. The uterus had, however, been almost twice as large approximately 2 weeks earlier. Not only did the uterus contract down, but also the central echoes of the uterus became smaller. These findings are compatible with incomplete, inevitable abortion.

Occasionally, the uterus will reach a fairly large size. If an abortion is present, degeneration of the fetus and placenta will occur. Often, this may be difficult to distinguish from a molar pregnancy. Figure 30 is a transverse scan of a patient with an incomplete abortion. The uterus is markedly enlarged. Diffuse, irregular echoes within it could be confused with a molar pregnancy. We can often distinguish an incomplete abortion from a molar pregnancy by the strong echoes present in an incomplete abortion.

Figure 31 is a longitudinal scan on the same patient demonstrating numerous strong echoes (arrows) within the uterus. This uneven echo pattern is highly suggestive of an inevitable abortion, rather than a molar pregnancy. Figure 32 further confirms this diagnosis, since calcification is noted within the uterus. That this is a calcific density is confirmed by the shadow distal to it. If such strong calcific echoes can be identified, the diagnosis of an inevitable abortion, as opposed to a molar pregnancy, can be made.

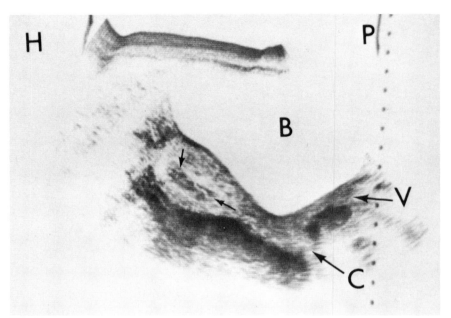

Fig. 29

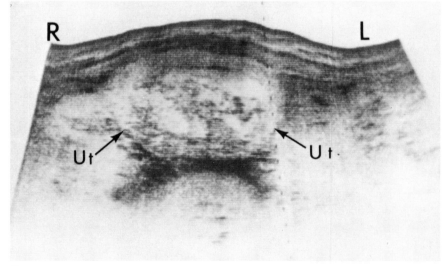

Fig. 30

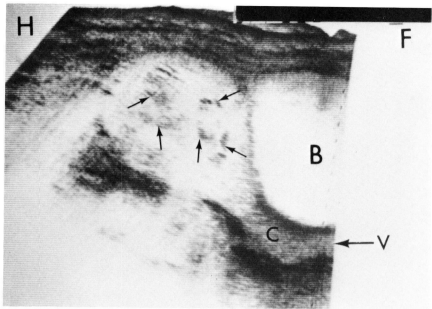

Arrows = Retained products of conception
B = Urinary bladder
C = Cervix
Ca = Calcification
H = Head
L = Left
P = Level of the symphysis pubis
R = Right
Sh = Shadowing
Ut = Uterus
V = Vagina

Fig. 31

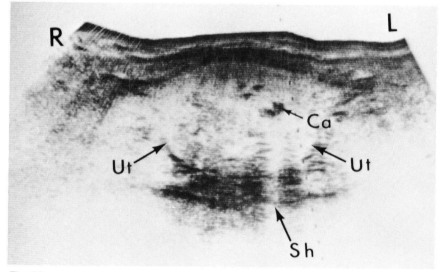

Fig. 32

Gestational Age

During the course of a pregnancy, several anatomic structures can be measured, all of which will give a fairly accurate assessment of gestational age. In the first 10 weeks of pregnancy, the gestational sac is used to measure the length of pregnancy. A mean gestational diameter is used by taking height, width, and length measurements and dividing these by three. Figure 33 is a longitudinal scan with the gestational sac seen in the central portion of the uterus. We can obtain a length and a height of the gestational sac, corresponding to the dark lines seen in figure 33. By obtaining a transverse scan and measuring the width, we can then determine the mean gestational sac diameter. This can be used from the fifth to the tenth menstrual week.

After the disappearance of the gestational sac, it is difficult to visualize the biparietal diameter for several weeks. During this period of time, the crown–rump length can be used to determine the gestational age. Crown rump length is often used from the seventh to the fifteenth or sixteenth menstrual week. Figure 34 is an example of the crown–rump length measured from the top of the fetal skull (number 1) to the sacral region (number 2).

The biparietal diameter is used to estimate gestational age from the fifteenth week of gestation to term. This diameter can occasionally be seen as early as the eleventh or twelfth week of gestation. By the fifteenth or sixteenth week, we should be able to obtain a biparietal diameter in 100% of cases. Figure 35 is a transverse scan of the fetal skull with a strong central linear echo which arises from the falx cerebri. On each side of the falx cerebri are some lucent areas arising from the lateral ventricles. When visualizing the lateral ventricles, we are too cephalad to obtain an accurate biparietal diameter. The biparietal diameter should be measured at the widest diameter of the fetal skull, which is at the level of the thalami.

Dr. Michael Johnson of the University of Colorado, Denver, Colorado, has recently developed newer concepts in understanding the anatomy of the fetal

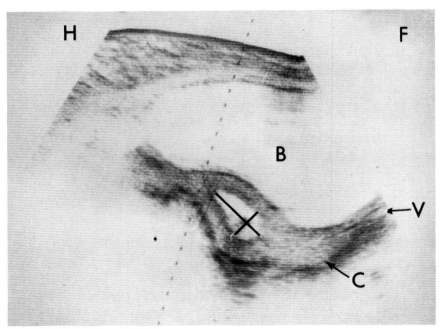

Fig. 33

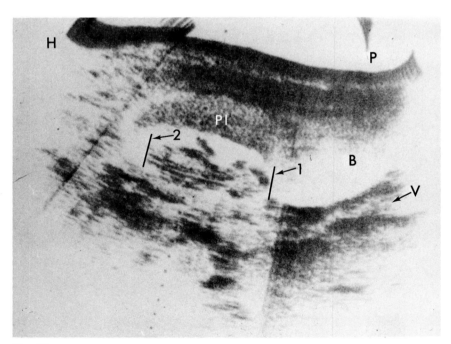

Fig. 34

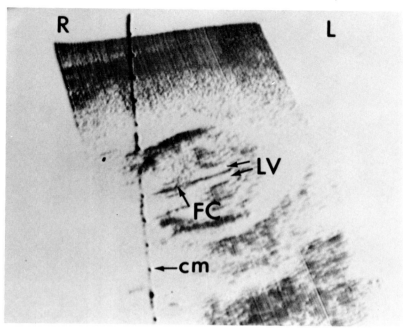

Fig. 35

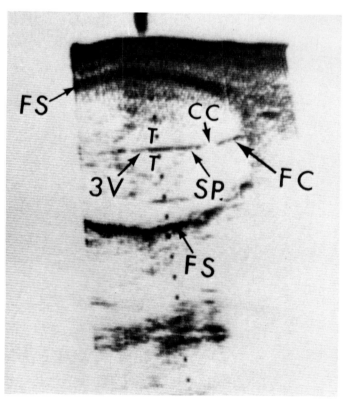

Fig. 36

skull. He has determined that the most accurate measurements for biparietal diameters are obtained at the level of the thalami. Figure 36 is a transverse scan of the fetal skull with the sonolucencies of the thalami situated near the central portion of the brain. The strong central echo between the thalami is arising from the third ventricle (number 3V). The continuation of the linear echo of the third ventricle arises from the septum pellucidum. A break is seen in the midline structures as the corpus callosum crosses the midline. The linear echoes then continue anteriorly formed by the falx cerebri. The biparietal diameter can then be obtained when visualizing the thalamic level. The biparietal diameters are measured from the near fetal skull to the far fetal skull.

B	=	Urinary bladder
C	=	Cervix
CC	=	Corpus callosum
cm	=	centimeter markers
F	=	Foot
FC	=	Falx cerebri
FS	=	Fetal skull
H	=	Head
L	=	Left
LV	=	Lateral ventricles
Numbers		
1 and 2	=	Crown–rump length (fig. 34)
Number		
3V	=	Third ventricle
P	=	Symphysis pubis
Perpendic-		
ular lines	=	Length and height of the gestational sac (fig. 33)
PL	=	Placenta
R	=	Right
SP	=	Septum pellucidum
T	=	Thalami
V	=	Vagina

Normal Placenta   I.

Placental tissue will present either as an echogenic area or as a sonolucent area, depending upon its position in relationship to the fetus and to the transducer. If an anterior placenta is present in which there are only the uterine and abdominal walls between the placenta and the transducer, it will present as an evenly speckled, echogenic area. Figure 37 is an example of an anterior placenta with an even, soft echogenic appearance to it. A strong linear echo between the placenta and the amniotic fluid is arising from the chorionic plate. Since the chorionic plate is a specular reflector, we must be close to the perpendicular in order to visualize the chorionic plate. It is not unusual to scan over an anterior placenta and, because of this physical limitation, be unable to visualize the chorionic plate. Figure 38 is another midline longitudinal scan with a homogeneous echo pattern arising from the anterior placenta. The placenta has an even texture with no masses evident within it. Mature placentas later on in pregnancy will tend to give an uneven coarser echo appearance.

Figures 39 and 40 are placentas with some small sonolucencies situated just beneath the chorionic plate. These are secondary to choriol cysts. They are a normal anatomic variant and of no clinical significance. Their usual location is directly beneath the chorionic plate.

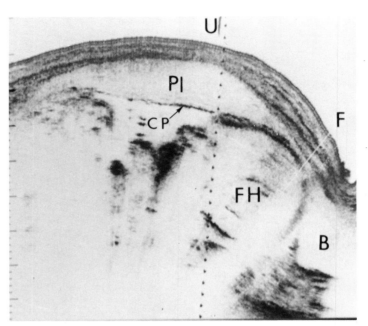

Fig. 37

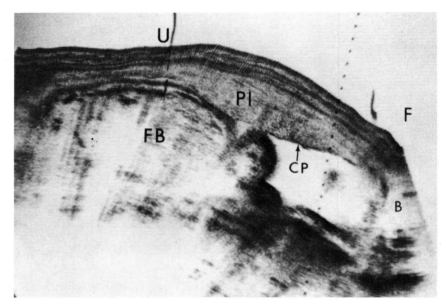

Fig. 38

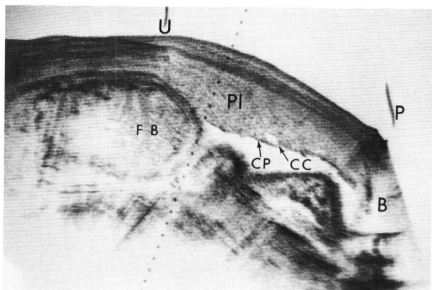

Fig. 39

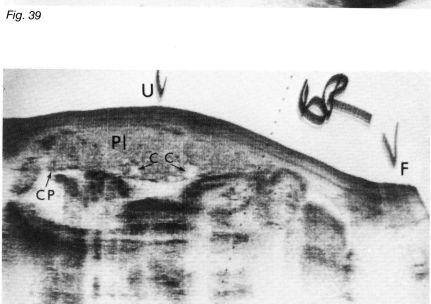

Fig. 40

Normal Placenta II.

When the placenta is situated posteriorly, it can give a variety of echogenic appearances. If it is situated behind the fetus, it will appear as a sonolucent area. The reason for this is that the echoes arising from the placenta are too weak to pass through the markedly attenuating osseous structures of the fetus. Therefore, the echoes are not registered on the transducer during their return from the placental interfaces. Figure 41 is an example of a longitudinal scan in which we have a posterior fundal placenta. Placental tissue in the fundal region deep to amniotic fluid is speckling in, much as the anterior placentas did on the previous scans. The intervening amniotic fluid does not attenuate the placental tissue. The placenta, however, is also situated deep to the fetal extremities and the fetal head. Placental tissue in this location appears as a sonolucent area because of the attenuation from the fetus.

Figure 42 is another example of echogenic placental tissue deep to amniotic fluid. Areas of placental shadowing, however, are noted when the placenta is scanned deep to the fetal extremities. There is a small region of through transmission as we scan between the fetal extremities. This is an extremely important technical concept to understand, because the limits of a posterior placenta are often quite difficult to detect.

Figure 43 is a transverse scan of a posterior lateral placenta with shadowing deep to the fetal body and fetal extremities. The left lateral portion of the placenta is seen. Here we have excellent visualization of the placental myometrial interface (arrows). The placental tissue is higher in amplitude and has a much finer echo appearance than the surrounding myometrium.

Figure 44 is a transverse scan of a posterior placenta. The placental tissue echoes normally when it is deep to the amniotic fluid on the left side. However, echogenicity from the placenta on the right side is also visualized when it is deep to the fetal body. The placenta was actually scanned from the right lateral aspect of the maternal abdomen. There-

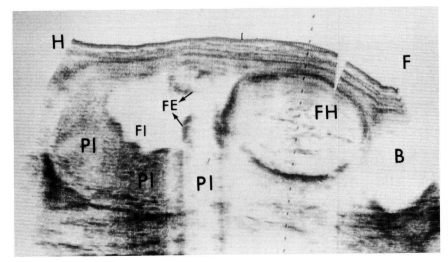

Fig. 41

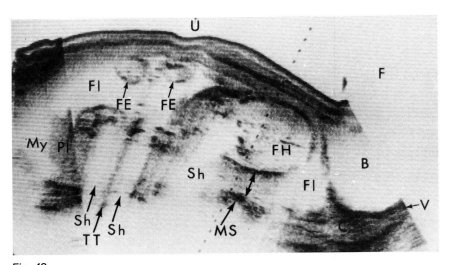

Fig. 42

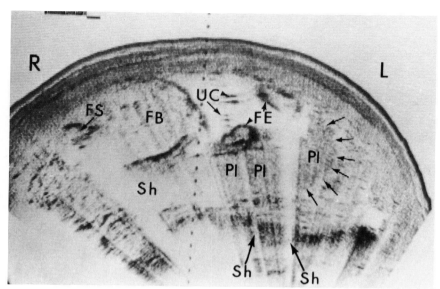

Fig. 43

fore, we did not pass the sound beam through the fetal body in order to speckle in the placenta on the right side. If we had scanned this patient from the anterior right abdomen, the placenta would have appeared sonolucent because of fetal body attenuation. The difference in echogenicity between the myometrium and placenta can be noted.

Arrows = Placental myometrial interface
(fig. 43)
B   = Urinary bladder
Ce = Cervix
F   = Foot
FB = Fetal body
FE = Fetal extremity
FH = Fetal head
FI = Amniotic fluid
FS = Fetal spine
H   = Head
L   = Left
MS = Maternal sacrum
My = Myometrium
Pl = Placenta
R   = Right
Sh = Shadowing
TT = Through transmission
U   = Umbilical level
UC = Umbilical cord
V   = Vagina

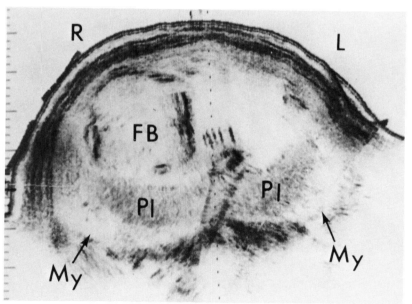

Fig. 44

Normal Placenta   III.

A fundal placenta usually yields echogenicity similar to an anterior placenta when no fetus is situated between the placenta and the transducer. Figure 45 is an example of the fundal posterior placenta. The echogenic portion of the placenta is visualized in the fundal region. The sonolucent myometrium is noted cephalad to the placental tissue. When we are scanning over the fetal body, however, the placenta, situated deep to the fetus, appears as a sonolucent mass. A transverse scan through a fundal placenta (fig. 46) demonstrates an even echo pattern to the placental tissue surrounded by the relatively more lucent myometrium. If we were to scan the entire uterus and this picture were obtained, a hydatidiform mole would be considered. Scanning a placenta tangentially, however, can give an appearance similar to figure 46.

There has been much discussion about placental migration and the disappearance of a placenta previa with time. This has been attributed by many to the fact that the myometrium grows at a differential rate compared to placental tissue. Another important point that must be understood, however, is that the uterus undergoes contractions during the course of many ultrasonic examinations. Figures 47 and 48 are excellent examples of uterine contraction apparently changing the placental location.

Figure 47 is a midline scan with an anterior placenta which is somewhat low-lying. The difference in echogenicity between the placenta and myometrium is noted. The arrows in figure 47 represent the placental myometrial interface. The patient was then scanned approximately 5 minutes later after slight emptying of the bladder. The following scan (fig. 48) indicates the anterior placenta to be no longer low-lying. The myometrium in figure 47 is also much thicker in the anterior lower uterine segment than that in figure 48. This represents a uterine contraction drawing the placenta closer to the endocervical canal in figure 47. With relaxation of the contraction (fig. 48), the placenta moves much more cephalad.

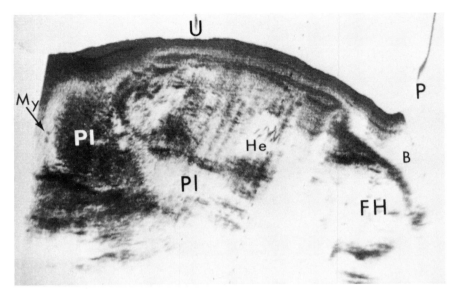

Fig. 45

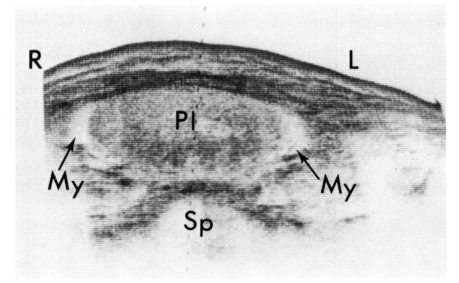

Fig. 46

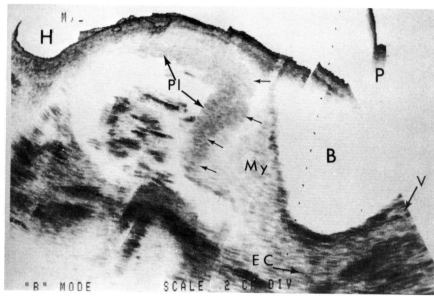

Fig. 47

Arrows	=	Placental myometrial inter-face (figs. 47 and 48)
B	=	Urinary bladder
EC	=	Endocervical canal
FH	=	Fetal head
H	=	Head
He	=	Fetal heart
L	=	Left
My	=	Myometrium
P	=	Symphysis pubis
Pl	=	Placenta
R	=	Right
Sp	=	Maternal spine
U	=	Umbilical level
V	=	Vagina

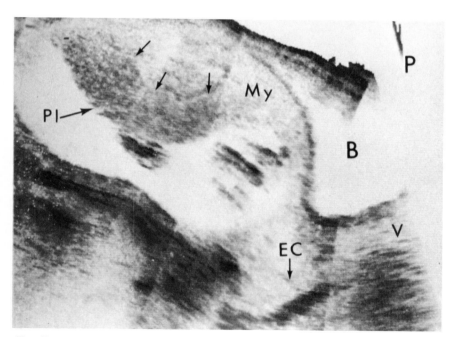

Fig. 48

Placental Myometrial Interface; Mature Placenta

When examining the placenta in a longitudinal or transverse plane, numerous tubular sonolucencies are often seen situated deep to it. In reality, this represents the myometrium with its rich vascular bed supplying the placenta. Figures 49 and 50 are longitudinal and transverse scans in which we see a markedly lucent and tubular myometrium deep to the placental tissues. This is not always a constant finding. In many individuals the myometrial-placental interface is not as dramatic as in these cases. When these marked tubular structures are present, however, they represent a normal variant with venous lakes within the myometrium standing out more prominently than usual. This should not be misdiagnosed as an abnormality or myometrial bleed. It does not represent an abruptio placenta, but rather a normal variant. Numerous parallel lines which represent the umbilical cord are also noted in figure 49. This is a normal finding on obstetrical examinations.

After the thirty-third or thirty-fourth week of pregnancy, many placentas will have an echogenic pattern different from the usual, even parenchymagram noted earlier in pregnancy. The appearance of the placenta will be much coarser and irregular. This is secondary to placental aging, which is a normal occurrence later on in pregnancy. Figure 51 is a longitudinal scan with a placenta with an even echo pattern in certain areas. Other areas, however, have very strong curvilinear echoes (arrows) that even cast a shadow. This is secondary to placental fibrosis and may eventually lead to placental calcification. Figure 52 is another longitudinal scan through the placenta. Multiple circular sonolucent areas represent the cotyledons of the placenta. These are surrounded by strong, highly echogenic rims (arrows) that represent areas of fibrosis and calcification. If we see this type of pattern earlier in pregnancy, around 27 weeks, we should be concerned about premature placental maturation.

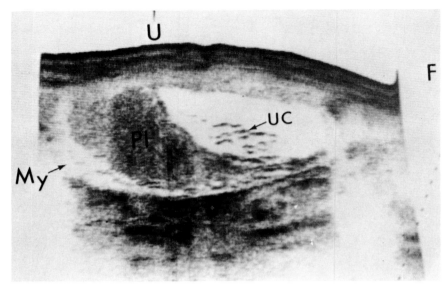

Fig. 49

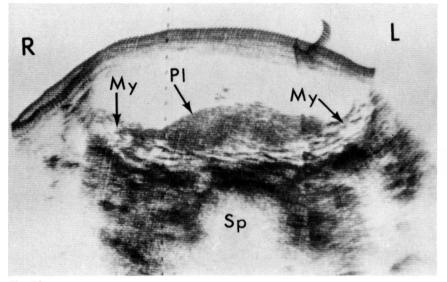

Fig. 50

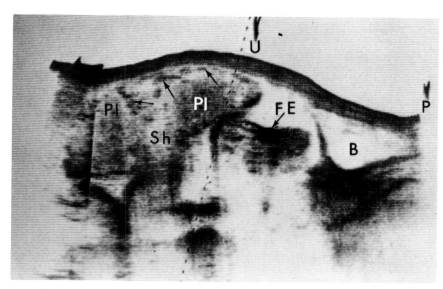

Arrows = Areas of placental fibrosis and calcification
B = Urinary bladder
Co = Placental cotyledons
F = Foot
FE = Fetal extremity
H = Head
L = Left
My = Myometrium
P = Level of the symphysis pubis
Pl = Placenta
R = Right
Sh = Shadowing
Sp = Spine
U = Umbilical level
UC = Umbilical cord

Fig. 51

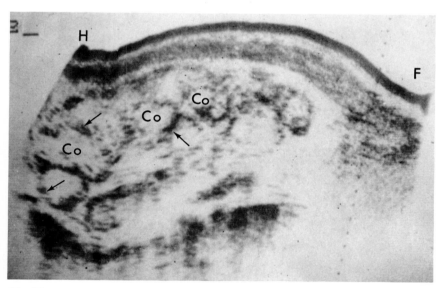

Fig. 52

Placenta Previa   I.

In examining a third-trimester bleeder for placenta previa, it is extremely important to visualize not only the cervix but also the endocervical canal. Figure 53 is a longitudinal scan with the strong linear echo of the endocervical canal seen within the myometrial echoes of the cervix. Since the cervix is quite wide, we can scan over a 4-cm area and just visualize the cervical myometrium without visualizing the endocervical canal. An important measurement in ruling out a posterior placenta previa is visualization of the distance between the fetal head and the maternal sacrum. In figure 53 the distance between the fetal head and maternal sacrum (small arrows) is only about 1 cm. This is in the normal range, since anything less than 1.6–2 cm is considered within normal limits. Figure 54 is another longitudinal scan with a normal distance between the fetal head and maternal sacrum. Again, it is extremely important to visualize the linear echo of the endocervical canal, which is well seen in figure 54.

Figure 55 is an example of an increased distance between the fetal head and maternal sacrum. In this instance it is approximately 3 cm. When the fetal head is elevated above the maternal sacrum, the possibility of a posterior previa should be considered. Other causes for the elevation of the fetal head include an extremity interposed between the fetal head and the maternal sacrum, or a fetal head that is off center, causing us to scan a lateral aspect that will appear to be elevated off the maternal sacrum. Whenever there is any question, it is important to have the patient continue filling her bladder and to make strong efforts to visualize the endocervical canal.

Figure 56 is an example of a bladder filled adequately enough to allow visualization of the endocervical canal. The placenta extends completely over the cervix on this scan. The placental-myometrial interface (arrows) is well seen on this study. When attempting to diagnose a posterior placenta previa, it is extremely important to visualize not only the cervix but also the endocervical

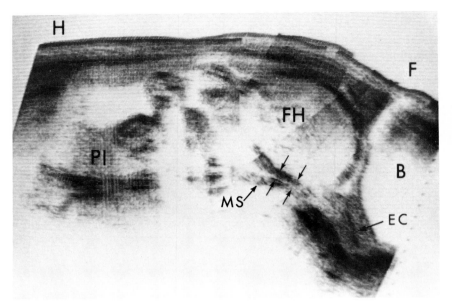

Fig. 53

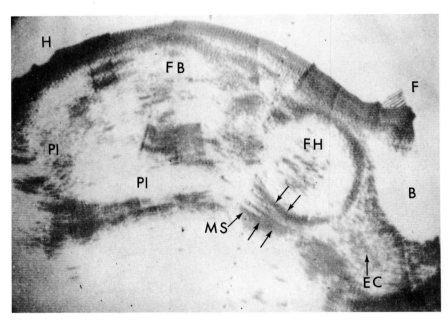

Fig. 54

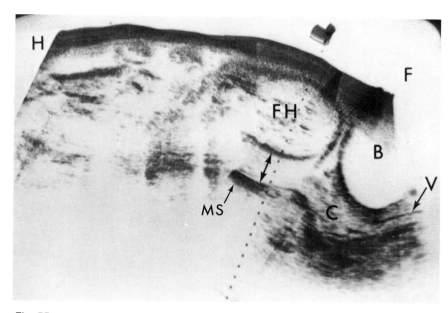

Fig. 55

canal and the placental myometrial interface, as is seen in figure 56. If this placental-myometrial interface can be seen extending over the entire cervix, the diagnosis of posterior placenta previa can be made.

Arrows	=	Fetal head-maternal sacral distance
Arrows	=	Placental-myometrial interface (fig. 56)
B	=	Urinary bladder
C	=	Cervix
EC	=	Endocervical canal
F	=	Foot
FB	=	Fetal body
FH	=	Fetal head
H	=	Head
MS	=	Maternal sacrum
PI	=	Placenta
V	=	Vagina

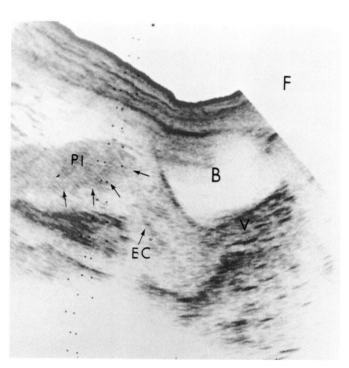

Fig. 56

Placenta Previa   II.

A central previa exists when the placenta is situated over the mid portion of the cervix with an equal component over the anterior myometrium and an equal component over the posterior myometrium. We are near the midline, since we are able to visualize the cervix on this scan (fig. 57). The placental-myometrial interface (arrows) is well visualized as a relatively lucent band caudal to the placenta itself. This is consistent with a central placenta previa.

Figure 58 is a longitudinal scan with a central previa with a large anterior component. Again we see the placental tissue situated over the endocervical canal. This is a complete previa, since placental tissue is situated both anterior and posterior to the cervix. When we see this much placenta over the endocervical canal, we should have no difficulty in diagnosing a placenta previa.

Figures 59 and 60 are examples of placenta previa with sonolucent areas also visualized within the placenta. In figure 59 we see a sonolucent area secondary to hemorrhage situated just beneath the chorionic plate of the placenta. This is a complete posterior previa, since placental tissue is seen over the cervix and endocervical canal. In figure 60 longitudinal scan demonstrates not only a posterior placenta previa, but also a small lucency separating the placenta from the cervix. This is a posterior previa with a sonolucent area situated between the placenta and cervix, corresponding to the area of hemorrhage.

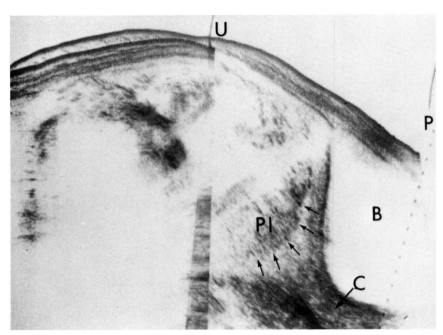

Fig. 57

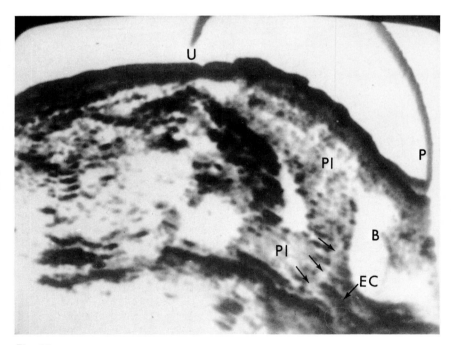

Fig. 58

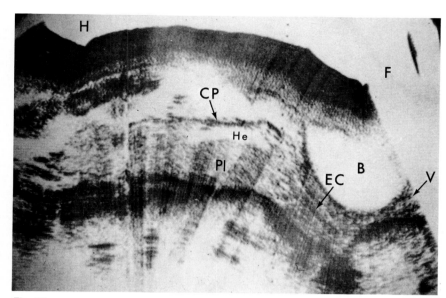

Fig. 59

SOURCE: The case in figure 58 is provided through the courtesy of Dr. M. Shaub, Centinela Valley Hospital, Los Angeles, California.

Arrows	=	Placental myometrial interface
B	=	Urinary bladder
C	=	Cervix
CP	=	Chorionic plate
Ec	=	Endocervical canal
F	=	Foot
Fe	=	Fetus
H	=	Head
He	=	Area of hemorrhage
P	=	Level of symphysis pubis
Pl	=	Placenta
U	=	Umbilical level
V	=	Vagina

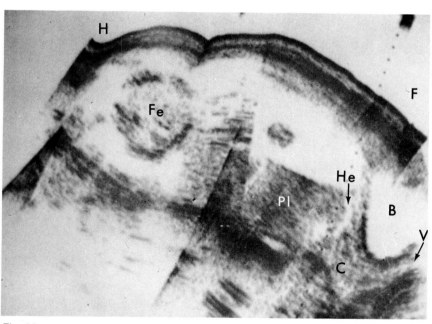

Fig. 60

Thick Placenta; Uterine Hematoma

Five centimeters is considered the upper limits for normal placental thickness. Several clinical entities can cause an increase in placental volume and thickness. The most common is Rh sensitization. Increase in placental thickness, however, can also be seen in diabetes and syphilis.

Figures 61 and 62 demonstrate examples of extreme placental thickness in a patient who had Rh sensitization with placental and fetal findings. Here we see marked thickness to the placenta, which is taking up the majority of the volume of the uterus. Figure 61 is a longitudinal scan in which only a portion of the fetal head is visualized, while the remainder of the uterine volume is filled with the placenta. Figure 62 is a transverse scan showing not only a thickened placenta but also ascites within the fetal abdomen. The fetal bowel is displaced away from the fetal abdominal wall. Only a small amount of amniotic fluid is present on this scan. This was true throughout the rest of this study. Practically the entire uterus is placenta-filled. Not only is the placenta markedly thickened in Rh sensitization, but it also has a high amplitude echogenicity.

Figures 63 and 64 are scans of an unusual patient with an area of hemorrhage in the cervical region of the uterus. Figure 63 is a longitudinal scan obtained on the patient on the same day that she suffered injuries in an auto accident. A sonolucent mass over the cervical region was suspected to be a uterine hematoma. The patient was followed for several weeks, and figure 64 is a study performed approximately 3–4 weeks after the previous examination. The uterine hematoma has completely resolved, and no sonolucent mass is evident in the lower uterine segment. This is an example of hemorrhage within the myometrium with complete resolution.

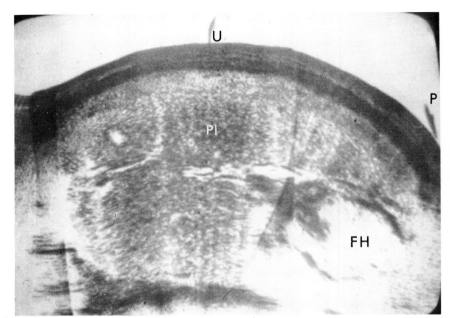

Fig. 61

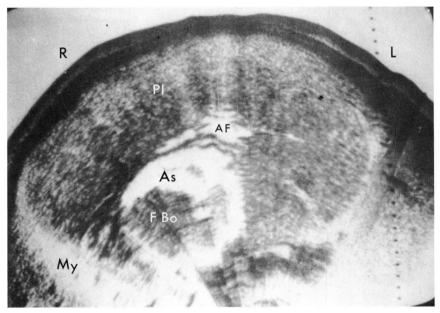

Fig. 62

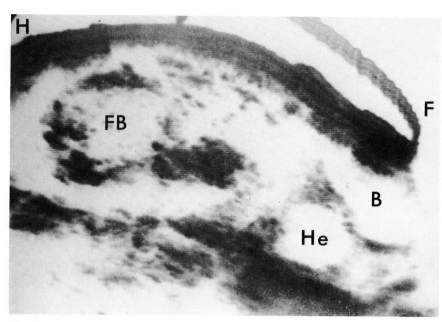

SOURCE: The case in figures 63 and 64 was provided through the courtesy of Dr. M. Shaub, Centinela Valley Hospital, Los Angeles, California.

AF	=	Amniotic fluid
As	=	Fetal ascites
B	=	Bladder
F	=	Foot
FB	=	Fetal body
FBo	=	Fetal bowel
FH	=	Fetal head
H	=	Head
He	=	Uterine hematoma
L	=	Left
My	=	Myometrium
P	=	Level of the symphysis pubis
Pl	=	Placenta
R	=	Right
U	=	Umbilical level

Fig. 63

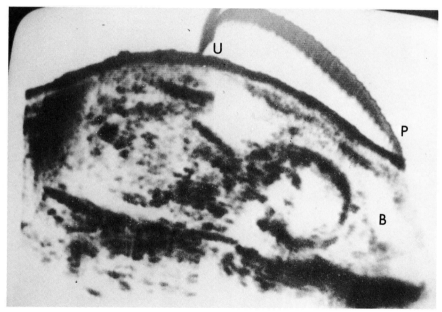

Fig. 64

Placental Implantation on a Uterine Septum

Occasionally during the course of an ultrasound examination we come across a placenta that has an unusual configuration. Figure 65 is an example of a 23-year-old woman with a confusing routine obstetrical ultrasound examination. On closer scrutiny of the study, however, a placental implantation on a uterine septum was diagnosed (fig. 65). In the center of figure 65 is a drawing which represents the findings at cesarean section. The fetus is in the breech position with the placenta implanted on a uterine septum. The fetal head is noted left of the placenta with the left arm situated on the right side of the uterine septum.

Part A of figure 65 is a transverse scan, quite cephalad with the fetal head on the left side of the uterus, to the left of the placenta. The placenta is situated against the lateral uterine wall on the right side. A transverse scan at part B shows that the placenta is now displaced away from the lateral uterine wall in which we see a sonolucent area of fluid. More caudally in part C of figure 65, we see the fetal extremity situated to the right lateral aspect of the placenta. The fetal body is situated to the left side. Part D is most important, for we are able to actually see the tip of the placenta as it extends into the amniotic fluid. The fetal extremity is visualized underneath the placenta with the fetal body to the left side.

Longitudinal scans corresponding to parts F, G, H, and I confirm the finding of a placental septum with the fetal extremity situated below the placenta and the fetal head and body situated on the left side. Cesarean section was performed on the patient and the findings corresponded to the initial ultrasonic interpretation.

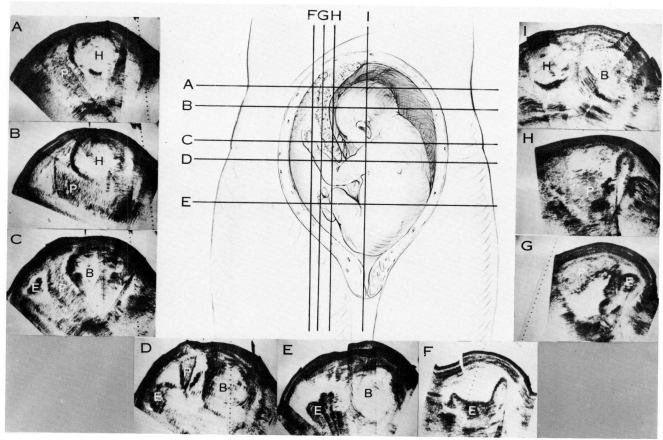

Fig. 65

B = Fetal body
E = Fetal extremity
H = Fetal head
P = Placenta

Multiple Gestation   I.

One of the more common referral diagnoses for obstetrical ultrasound is that
the patient is too "large for dates." Most
often the reason for this discrepancy between size and dates is the fact that the
patient is unsure of her last menstrual
period. Another cause, however, is multiple gestation. In the first 10 weeks of
pregnancy, we may actually be able to
visualize two gestational sacs (fig.
66). This transverse scan demonstrates a septum (arrow) between the
two gestational sacs (numbers 1 and 2).
Later on in pregnancy, when attempting
to diagnose a multiple gestation, it is
important to visualize the two fetal
heads. Figure 67 is an example of
two fetuses in the vertex presentation.
Both fetal heads are seen.

In figure 68 we are able to visualize one fetal head and two areas of amniotic fluid (numbers 1 and 2). Between
the two areas of fluid is a linear echo
representing the septum between the
two amniotic fluid cavities. Figure 69
is another example with the linear echo
(arrow) separating the fetal body on one
side and the fetal pelvis on the other.

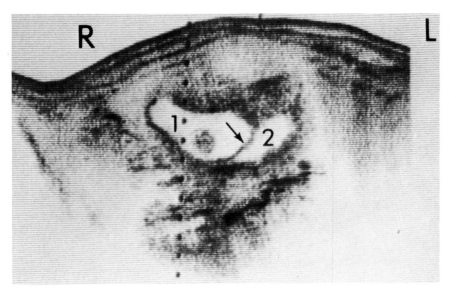

Fig. 66

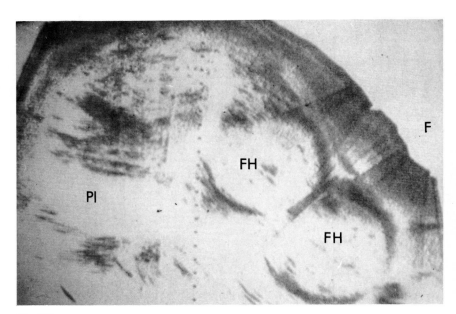

Fig. 67

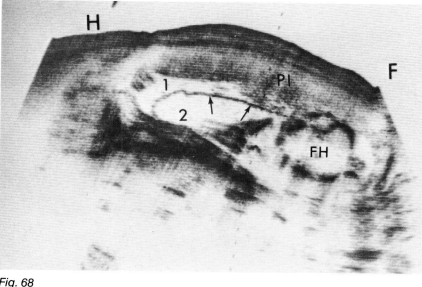

Arrows	=	Septum between the amniotic sacs
F	=	Foot
FH	=	Fetal head
FP	=	Fetal pelvis
H	=	Head
L	=	Left
Numbers		
1 and 2	=	Separate gestational sacs in a twin pregnancy (fig. 66)
Numbers		
1 and 2	=	Amniotic fluid (fig. 68)
PI	=	Placenta
R	=	Right
st	=	Fetal stomach
uv	=	umbilical veins

Fig. 68

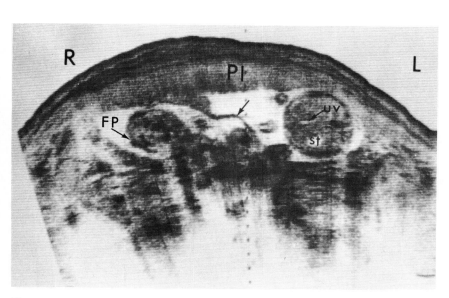

Fig. 69

Multiple Gestation II.

If several heads or bodies are present on ultrasound examination, the possibility of triplets should be considered. Most often, when several fetal heads are seen, the diagnosis of twins is made quite easily. An effort should be made, however, to map out the position of the fetuses on the patient's abdomen with a marking pencil. If carefully done, the diagnosis of triplets will not be missed. If we casually make the diagnosis of twins without attempting to determine the position of the fetus, however, we may miss triplets or quadruplets.

Figure 70 is a longitudinal scan with three fetal heads and one fetal body. When doing an examination on a patient who has a multiple gestation, it is extremely helpful to line up the fetal heads on one scan to confirm the number of fetuses present. On this scan, three of the fetal heads are aligned with one of the fetal bodies. Figure 71 demonstrates triplets with two fetal heads and one fetal body. We know, however, that the fetal body is separate from the two fetal heads because of the septum (arrows) separating the one fetal body from the two visualized fetal heads. The third fetal head was present much more caudally than this transverse cut.

Figures 72 and 73 are scans of another patient obtained several months apart. The initial scan was performed when the patient was at approximately 15–16 weeks' gestation. In figure 72 the transverse scan demonstrates a fetal head situated quite anteriorly. Suggestion of a second fetal head was noted in the posterior aspect of the uterus. This was approximately the same size as the first fetal head, and the possibility of twins was raised. The questionable fetal head, however, is situated posterior to the placenta and

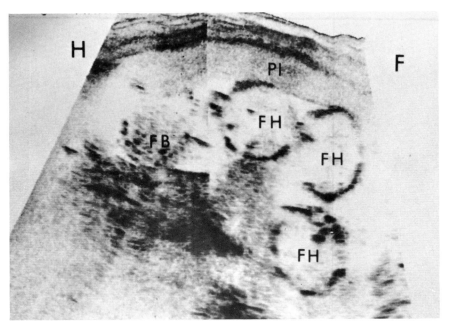

Fig. 70

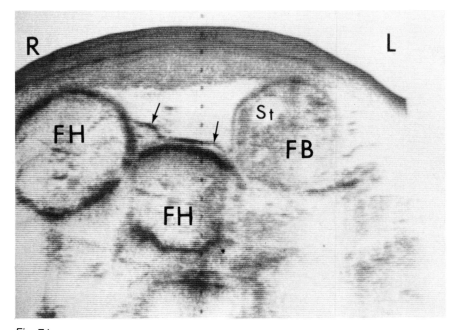

Fig. 71

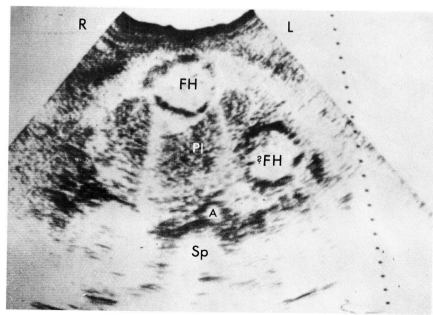

Fig. 72

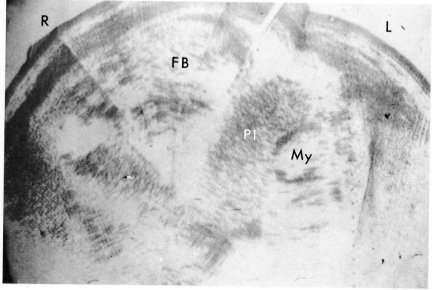

Fig. 73

actually in the myometrium. It was felt that this was a calcified myoma, which happened to be approximately the same size as the fetal head at 16 weeks' gestation. The patient was reexamined approximately 2 months later after adequate growth of fetal head and body. Figure 73 is a transverse scan in which a much larger fetal body is seen anterior to the placenta. The myoma is now visualized in the myometrium of the uterus posterior to the placenta. Therefore, the finding in figure 72 was a calcified myoma in the myometrium that just happened to have the appearance of a fetal head.

A	=	Aorta
Arrows	=	Septum separating the amniotic cavities
F	=	Foot
FB	=	Fetal body
FH	=	Fetal head
H	=	Head
L	=	Left
My	=	Calcified myoma
Pl	=	Placenta
R	=	Right
Sp	=	Spine
St	=	Stomach

Polyhydramnios

Another cause for the patient being "large for dates" is polyhydramnios. This is commonly caused by a slight imbalance between the mother and fetus, with no definite etiology arising from the fetus. Other causes which can be diagnosed by ultrasound are anencephaly and a high gastrointestinal obstruction in the fetus. When making the diagnosis of polyhydramnios, it is important to scan the entire uterus. We often can have one or two transverse scans or one longitudinal scan demonstrating a large amount of fluid; when the entire uterus is scanned, however, it will be realized that a normal amount of fluid is present. In the case of polyhydramnios, practically all scans demonstrate a large quantity of fluid.

Figures 74–77 are transverse and longitudinal scans of a patient with an anencephalic fetus. In every scan we see an inordinate amount of fluid. The amniotic fluid is markedly increased in quantity compared to the amount of fetal echoes visualized. The placenta is quite thin, due to pressure from the polyhydramnios. Only the fetal body can be visualized in this study. During the course of the entire examination, the fetal head was never identified. One sign of polyhydramnios is that fetal extremities are seen to be floating in the amniotic fluid on numerous scans. The amount of amniotic fluid is difficult to quantitate presently. Consequently, diagnosing polyhydramnios is still a subjective procedure. In the future we hope to be able to quantitate the amount of fluid present in the uterus.

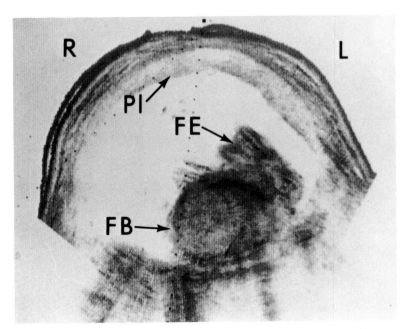

Fig. 74

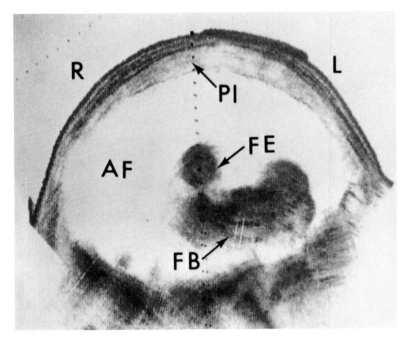

Fig. 75

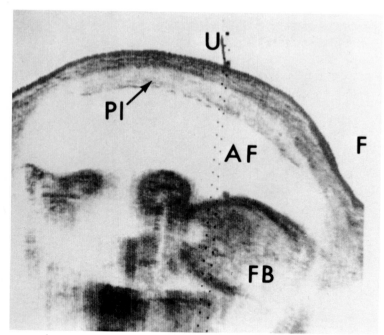

Fig. 76

AF = Amniotic fluid
F = Foot
FB = Fetal body
FE = Fetal extremity
L = Left
PI = Placenta
R = Right
U = Umbilicus

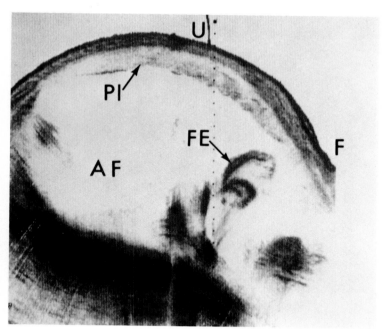

Fig. 77

Mass Associated with Pregnancy I.

Another reason for a patient referred to ultrasound as "large for dates" is a pelvic mass found in addition to a pregnancy. Often, a pelvic mass will elevate the uterus out of the pelvis, and clinically, the patient will appear to be "large for dates." One common mass seen during pregnancy is a corpus luteum cyst which supports the pregnancy for the first 4–5 months. Figure 78 is a longitudinal scan with a corpus luteum cyst situated in the cul-de-sac, elevating the fundus of the uterus to a higher position than is normally expected for the time of gestation. A gestational sac is situated in the fundus of the uterus.

Figure 79 is a longitudinal scan of a patient with an ovarian cyst above the fundus of the uterus. The ovarian cyst was actually palpated as the fundus of the uterus, and the patient was felt to be 6–8 weeks further along than she actually was. A gestational sac of approximately 7–8 weeks' gestation is seen. The top of the ovarian cyst, however, is approximately at the umbilical level, which would place this pregnancy at 16 weeks.

Figures 80 and 81 are transverse and longitudinal scans of a patient with a sonolucent mass in the right adnexal region. The pregnancy is situated in the midline and to the left of midline with the large sonolucent mass on the right side. The sonolucent mass has a strong linear echo in its posterior aspect indicating that this is not a simple cyst. It turned out to be a multilocular ovarian cyst that was quite large and also led to a "large-for-dates" discrepancy early on in the pregnancy.

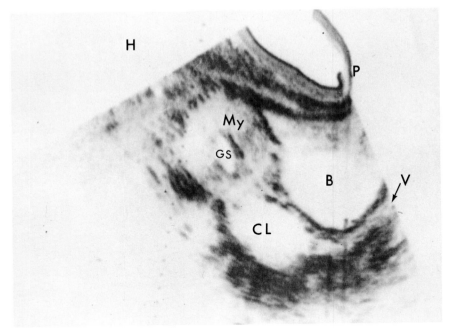

Fig. 78

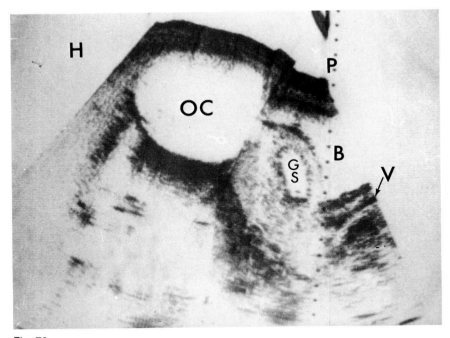

Fig. 79

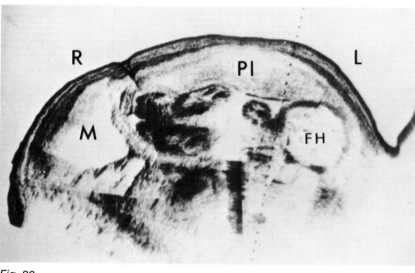

Fig. 80

B   = Urinary bladder
CL = Corpus luteum cyst
F   = Foot
FH = Fetal head
GS = Gestational sac
H   = Head
L   = Left
M   = Multiloculated ovarian cyst
My = Myometrium of the fundus of the
      uterus
OC = Ovarian cyst
P   = Level of the symphysis pubis
PI = Placenta
R   = Right
U   = Umbilical level
V   = Vagina

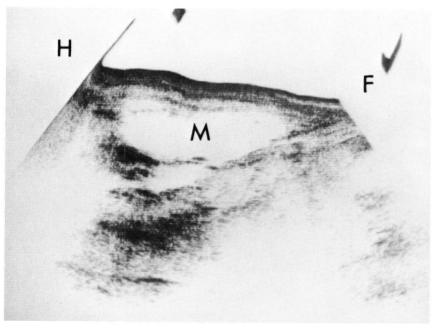

Fig. 81

Mass Associated with Pregnancy II.

Figure 82 is a longitudinal scan of a patient who also was considered to be "large for dates." We see a large sono-lucent mass situated in the lower pelvis posterior to the cervix. The cervix is elevated anteriorly. This was not the urinary bladder. The urinary bladder was completely empty on this longitudinal scan. At surgery, it was found to be a cystic teratoma situated in the cul-de-sac and markedly elevating the lower uterine segment anteriorly and cephaladly. The large size of the mass indicates that the fundus of the uterus would be elevated 6–8 cm higher than it normally would.

Frequently, the uterus itself may have a mass which causes it to be enlarged. Figure 83 demonstrates a small myoma in the posterior aspect of the uterus. A gestational sac is situated in the normal fundal position. Through transmission is posterior to the gestational sac, as the myometrium has increased echoes. The myoma elevates the uterus slightly and could give a mistaken diagnosis of an enlarged uterus.

Figure 84 is of another myomatous uterus with the fundal region of the uterus markedly more cephalad than it would be under normal circumstances. Here we see a gestational sac situated in the fundal region of the uterus. It is approximately 4 cm in diameter which would place it at 9–10 weeks. The myoma, however, is approximately 10–12 cm in diameter. This places the fundus of the uterus at approximately 24 weeks' gestation, rather than the expected 8 weeks according to the size of the gestational sac. This would yield a clinical diagnosis of a "large-for-dates" patient. The myoma has a thoroughly characteristic echo pattern with attenuation seen posteriorly.

Figure 85 is a transverse scan of an interesting patient with approximately 7 weeks' gestation, as demonstrated by the size of the gestational sac. A strong echogenic mass is situated anterior to the uterus. A cleavage plane is between the mass and the uterus. This turned out to be an ovarian neoplasm which gave the patient a "large-

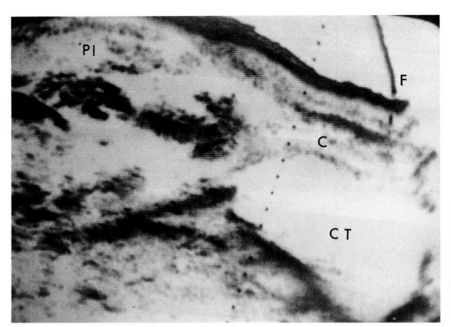

Fig. 82

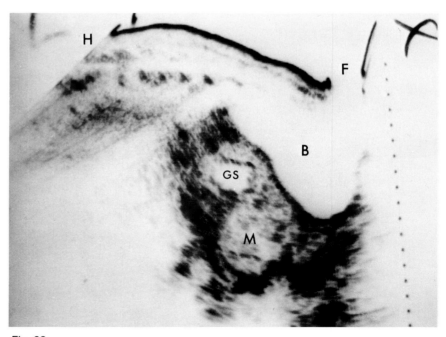

Fig. 83

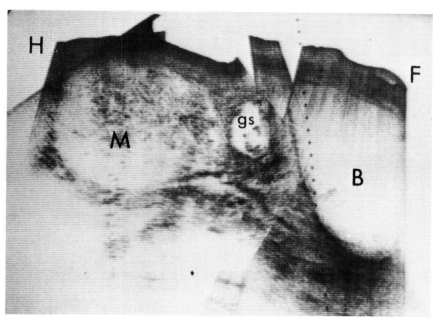

Fig. 84

left adnexal region is a small amount of fluid.

SOURCE: Figures 82 and 83 are provided through the courtesy of Dr. M. Shaub, Centinela Valley Hospital, Los Angeles, California.

B	=	Urinary bladder
C	=	Cervix
CT	=	Cystic teratoma
F	=	Foot
Fl	=	Fluid
GS	=	Gestational sac
gs	=	gestational sac
H	=	Head
L	=	Left
M	=	Neoplasm (fig. 84)
M	=	Myoma
Pl	=	Placenta
R	=	Right

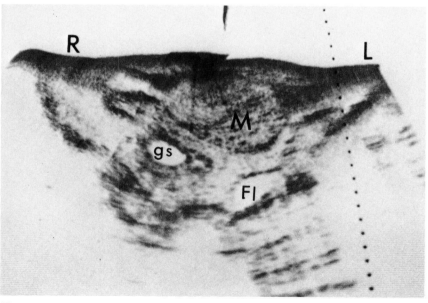

Fig. 85

Pelvic Kidney; Renal Transplant

Another cause for a "large-for-dates" referral, along with various masses in the pelvis, are ectopic kidneys or renal transplants. Figures 86 and 87 are scans of a pregnant woman with a pelvic kidney. The longitudinal scan (fig. 86) shows the kidney to be posterior to the fundal region of the uterus. The fetus is situated in the amniotic fluid with an anterior placenta. A transverse scan of the same patient is present in figure 87 with the kidney again seen posterior to the uterus.

Figures 88 and 89 are scans of a patient with a renal transplant in the right iliac fossa. Figure 88 is a transverse scan with a kidney situated in the right lateral abdomen lateral to the fetal head. A small amount of fluid is present within the kidney, secondary to mild hydronephrosis. Figure 89 is a longitudinal scan of the right lateral abdomen with the kidney situated in the lower right abdomen. Cephalad to the kidney, we see a relatively lucent echogenic region scanned tangentially through the myometrium of the uterus.

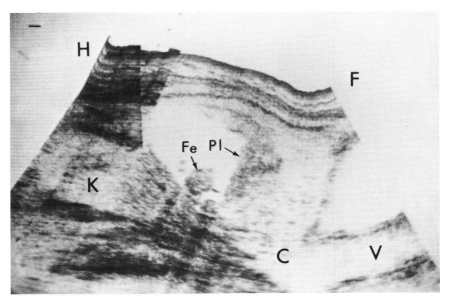

Fig. 86

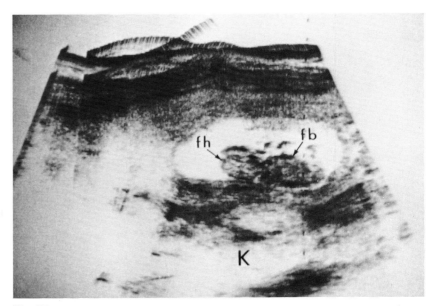

Fig. 87

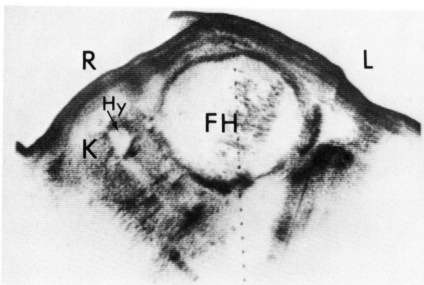

Fig. 88

B	=	Urinary bladder
C	=	Cervix
F	=	Foot
fb	=	Fetal body
Fe	=	Fetus
FH	=	Fetal head
fh	=	Fetal head
H	=	Head
Hy	=	Mild hydronephrosis
K	=	Pelvic kidney
K	=	Transplanted kidney (figs. 88 and 89)
L	=	Left
My	=	Myometrium
Pl	=	Placenta
R	=	Right
V	=	Vagina

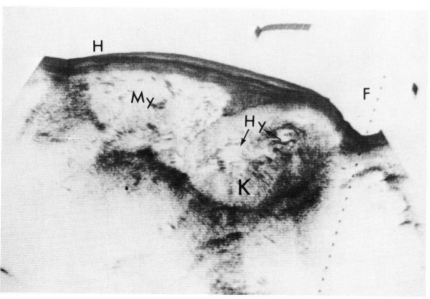

Fig. 89

Hydatidiform Mole

Yet another cause for a "large-for-dates" referral is a hydatidiform mole. In this instance, the fetus is felt to be at 16 or 18 weeks gestation, and no fetal heart tones are present. Usually, the clinician will request an ultrasound study to rule out fetal death. A hydatidiform mole gives a fairly characteristic echo pattern on ultrasound. Figures 90 and 91 are longitudinal and transverse scans of a patient with a molar pregnancy. Here we see a fairly even echo pattern throughout the uterus. The mole looks like placental tissue throughout. If, when scanning the uterus we find echogenicity of placental tissue throughout, the diagnosis of a molar pregnancy can be made.

Figures 92 and 93 are of another molar pregnancy within the confines of the uterus. Here we see some lucent structures indicating the larger grapelike structures within a hydatidiform mole. This type of molar pregnancy can be confused with a degenerated placenta and fetus. Even when scanning the uterus in its entirety, however, we do not find any calcific echoes or shadows when dealing with a molar pregnancy.

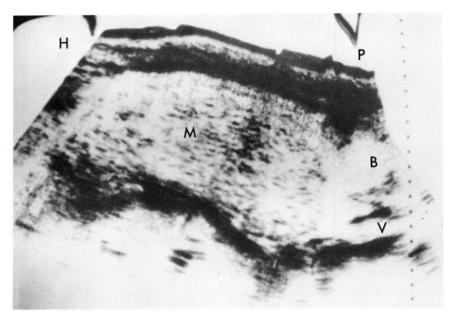

Fig. 90

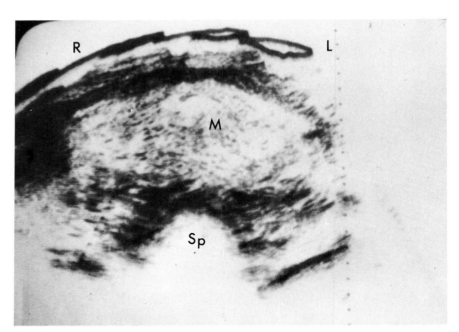

Fig. 91

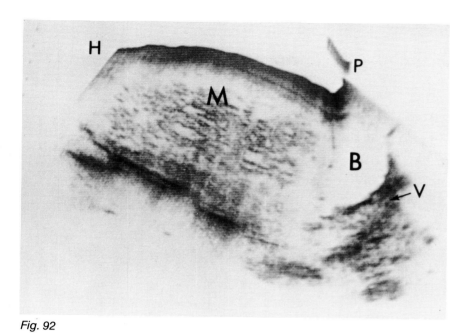

B = Urinary bladder
H = Head
L = Left
M = Hydatidiform mole
P = Level of the symphysis pubis
R = Right
Sp = Spine
V = Vagina

Fig. 92

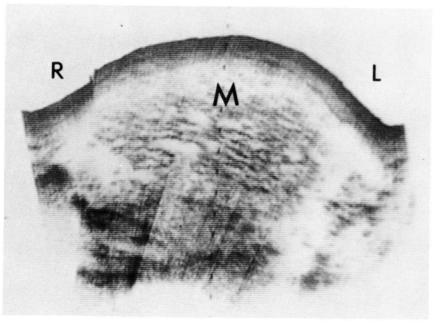

Fig. 93

Degenerating Placenta and Fetus

A hydatidiform mole can easily be confused for a degenerating pregnancy. Figures 94 and 95 are examples of early degeneration of the placenta (arrows). Numerous sonolucent structures are seen within the placental tissue. This is highly suggestive of a hydatidiform mole. In figure 94, however, we have enough amniotic fluid present, so there is no difficulty in distinguishing this as a pregnancy rather than a molar pregnancy. Figure 95 is a transverse scan with some remaining fetal echoes. When severe placental and fetal degeneration occurs, this picture can often be confused with a hydatidiform mole.

Figures 96 and 97 are of a degenerating pregnancy with some confusion as to whether or not we are dealing with a molar pregnancy. The longitudinal scan (fig. 96) demonstrates numerous strong echoes (arrows) throughout the uterus. A molar pregnancy usually has a fairly even echo pattern to it, more consistent with placental tissue. A degenerating pregnancy, as in this case, tends to have a coarser echogenic appearance. Figure 97 is the same case. Several sonolucent areas (arrows) are dispersed throughout the uterus. We are usually able to determine a degenerating pregnancy because of the coarseness and unevenness of the echo pattern. A molar pregnancy has a rather even speckled appearance to it. Because of the spectrum, however, overlap of the two entities is possible. In some instances, distinguishing between the two can be quite difficult.

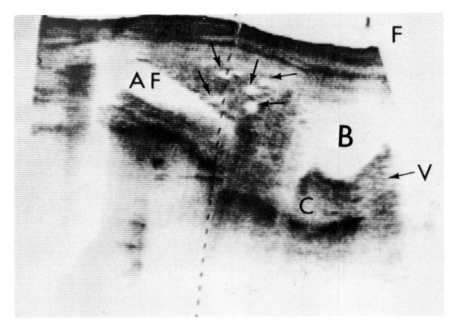

Fig. 94

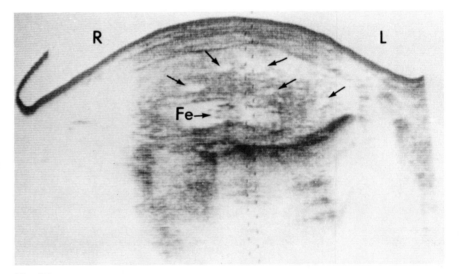

Fig. 95

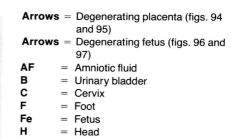

Arrows = Degenerating placenta (figs. 94
              and 95)
Arrows = Degenerating fetus (figs. 96 and
              97)
AF   = Amniotic fluid
B   = Urinary bladder
C   = Cervix
F   = Foot
Fe   = Fetus
H   = Head
L   = Left
R   = Right
Sp   = Spine
V   = Vagina

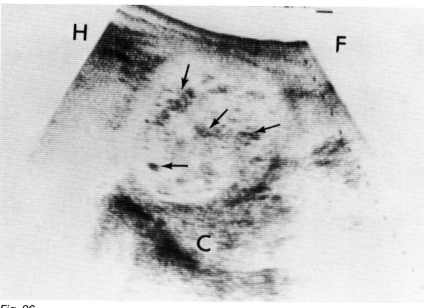

Fig. 96

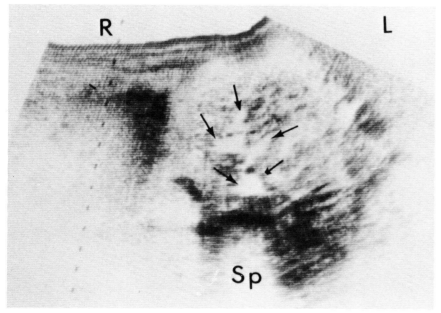

Fig. 97

Normal Fetal Anatomy   I.

When examining the obstetrical patient, it is important to pay particular attention to the anatomy of the fetus. While doing a routine obstetrical study, a great deal can be discovered about the normal anatomy. This becomes extremely important when examining the fetus for various congenital anomalies. Figure 98 is an example of a fetal head with fluid-filled lateral ventricles. Recognizing the normal lateral ventricles is extremely important when ruling out hydrocephalus. The lateral ventricles are much more easily visualized on real-time examination.

Frequently, an evaluation of the fetal spine for such entities as spina bifida or meningomyelocele is requested. Figure 99 is a longitudinal scan in which we see the tubular structure of the fetal spine. Shadowing is seen also over the thoracic region secondary to the fetal ribs.

Figure 100 is another of the fetal spine. In the region of the cervical spine, the fetal head and upper fetal spine are seen quite well. Posterior to the fetal spine is amniotic fluid. To rule out a meningocele or a meningomyelocele, close scrutiny of this cervical region would be ncessary. In following the fetal spine in a cephalad portion, a mass in the posterior cervical region can be ruled out. We can also scan the fetal spine in the lower sacral area to rule out any masses in this region. Figure 101 is a longitudinal scan in which the step-like echoes of the vertebral bodies are actually seen. The vertebral bodies yield this characteristic echo which can identify the fetal spinal column quite easily.

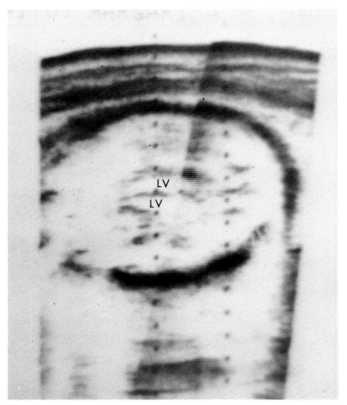

Fig. 98

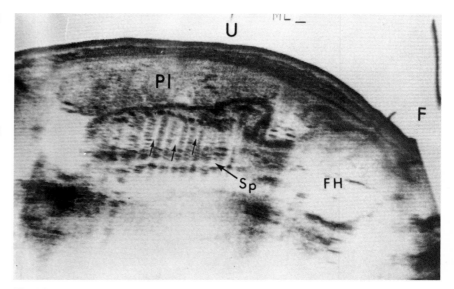

Fig. 99

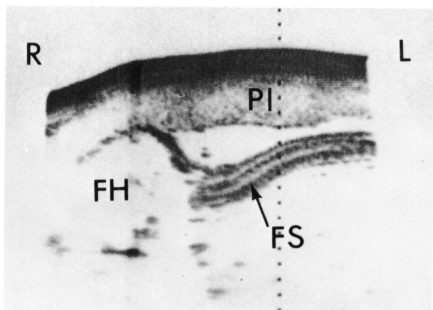

AF	= Amniotic fluid
Arrows	= Shadowing from the ribs
F	= Foot
FH	= Fetal head
FS	= Fetal spine
H	= Head
L	= Left
LV	= Lateral ventricles
Pl	= Placenta
R	= Right
Sp	= Fetal spine
U	= Umbilical level
Ve	= Vertebral bodies

Fig. 100

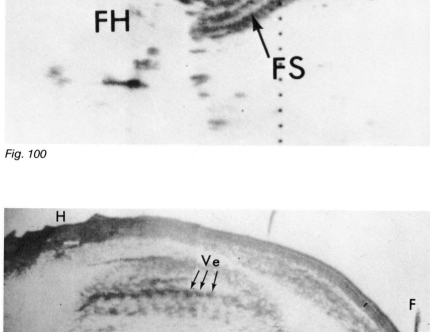

Fig. 101

Normal Fetal Anatomy   II.

Figure 102 is a transverse section of a fetus in the thoracic region. Here we see the fetal spine in a transverse plane. It appears as a circular echogenic region in the posterior aspect of the fetus. If a severe spina bifida were present, a defect would appear in the posterior aspect of the spine. A sonolucency is noted in the anterior half of the fetal thorax on this scan; this represents the fetal heart. By scanning slowly over the fetal cardiac region in either a transverse or longitudinal plane, fetal cardiac activity can be documented by B-scan. If there is any question at all, either Doppler or real time can be used to document fetal cardiac activity.

Figure 103 is a transverse scan over the fetal abdomen. Again we see the fetal spine in the posterior aspect of the fetal abdomen. A sonolucent area is present in the left upper quadrant; this is secondary to fluid in the fetal stomach. We can document fetal swallowing as fluid is recognized routinely in the fetal stomach. The linear tubular structure in the anterior half of the fetal abdomen is secondary to the umbilical vessels coursing through the fetal abdomen. This is an important landmark when attempting to measure the abdominal circumference of the fetus. Figure 104 is another transverse scan through the fetal abdomen with the fetal spine situated posteriorly. The left kidney is recognized posterior to the fetal stomach. Looking for renal abnormalities in utero, we can easily identify the fetal kidneys in the mid and third trimester.

Another transverse scan (fig. 105) allows both kidneys to be visualized this time. The left kidney is situated posterior to the fluid-filled fetal stomach again. In this instance, the fetal spleen is recognized lateral to the left kidney and fetal stomach. The paraspinous muscles are posterior to the kidneys.

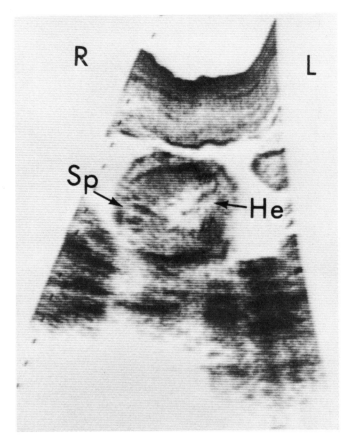

Fig. 102

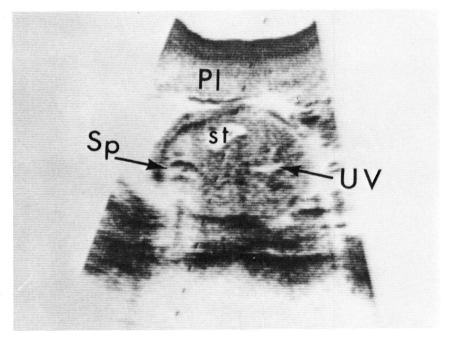

Fig. 103

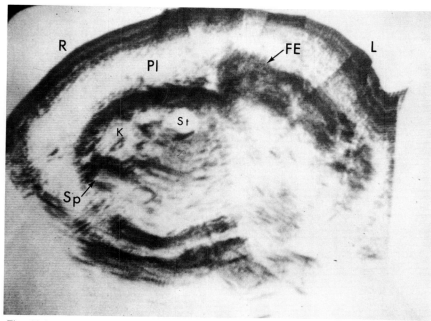

Fig. 104

FE	=	Fetal extremity
He	=	Fetal heart
K	=	Fetal kidneys
L	=	Left
Pl	=	Placenta
PM	=	Paraspinous muscles
R	=	Right
S	=	Spleen
Sp	=	Fetal spine
St	=	Fetal stomach
st	=	Stomach
UV	=	Umbilical vessels

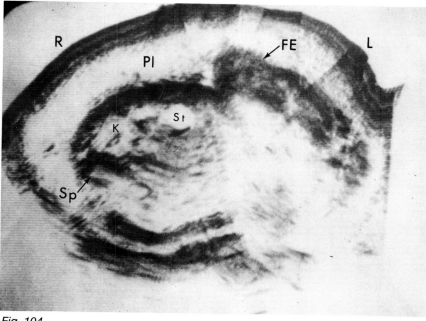

Fig. 105

Normal Fetal Anatomy   III.

Figure 106 is a coronal section of the fetus with the fetal heart in the thorax of the fetus. Just caudal to the fetal heart is the sonolucency of the stomach. This scan is an unusual one; the left kidney is visualized in the coronal plane. Figure 107 is another coronal section with the descending aorta just below the fetal heart. In this scan we are able to visualize both the right and left kidneys in a coronal section.

In figure 108 the thoracic and abdominal aorta is seen. The aorta in longitudinal scans presents as a small tubular structure. When scanning over the aorta at a rather slow rate, cardiac pulsations can actually be detected in the walls. The small size of the aorta in this scan is noted. The lumen is approximately 2 mm in diameter which demonstrates some of the resolution presently available with the various equipment. The mother often asks to know the sex of the baby. If the scan is successful, and the sex is evident, the scrotum may be detected. Figure 109 is a scan through the pelvis of the fetus; the urine-filled fetal bladder is seen. The scrotum is recognized in the amniotic fluid. Fetal urine production can be followed by measuring the volume of the fetal bladder at various intervals.

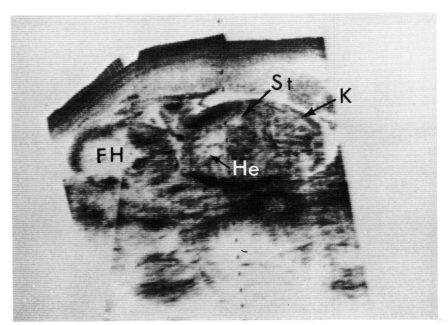

Fig. 106

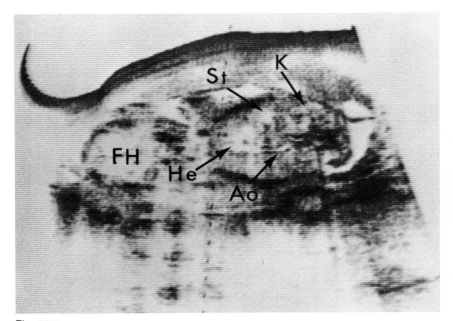

Fig. 107

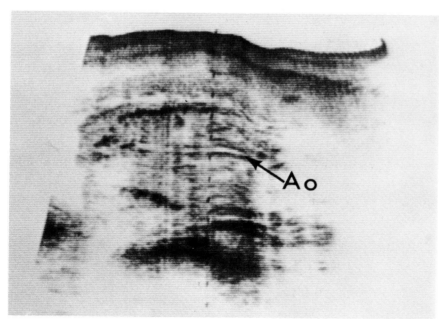

Ao = Aorta
FB = Fetal bladder
FH = Fetal head
He = Heart
K = Kidney
L = Left
R = Right
Sc = Scrotum
St = Stomach

Fig. 108

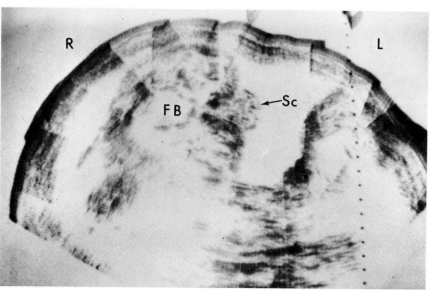

Fig. 109

Normal Fetal Anatomy   IV.

Figure 110 is a longitudinal scan over the lateral uterus with the characteristic echoes of a fetal extremity cut transversely. The fetal extremities yield a strong central echo arising from the osseous structure surrounded by the soft echoes of the muscle. Numerous parallel lines are noted on this scan. These are characteristic echoes arising from the umbilical cord. Figure 111 is a scan of the lower extremity of the fetus. The femur is situated in the thigh. Caudal to this, the tibia is visualized in the calf. The diagnosis of dwarfism may be possible with ultrasound when the osseous structures can be seen in such detail. Figure 112 is an excellent example of visualization of the upper extremity. The arm can be seen situated lateral to the fetal trunk. The strong echoes arising from the humerus are seen between the shoulder and fetal elbow. The forearm and digits of the hand can be seen quite well. Figure 113 is a well-known slide provided by Dr. Peter Cooperberg. It expresses most aptly the feeling of the majority of fetuses to ultrasonic probing. In reality, it is bowel loops surrounded by ascites.

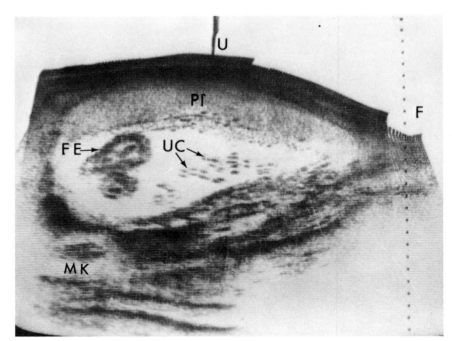

Fig. 110

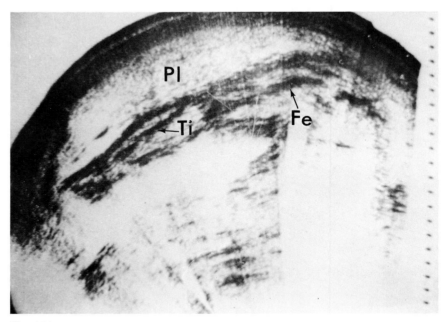

Fig. 111

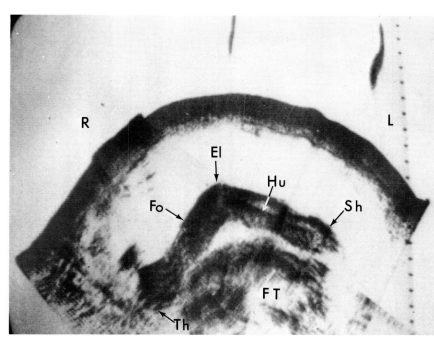

Fig. 112

Source: Figure 113 is provided through the courtesy of Dr. P. Cooperberg, University of British Columbia, Vancouver, British Columbia, Canada.

El	=	Elbow
F	=	Foot
FE	=	Fetal extremity
Fe	=	Femur
Figure 113	=	Bowel loops in ascites
Fo	=	Forearm
FT	=	Fetal trunk
Hu	=	Humerus
L	=	Left
MK	=	Maternal kidney
Pl	=	Placenta
R	=	Right
Sh	=	Shoulder
Th	=	Thumb
Ti	=	Tibia
U	=	Umbilical level
UC	=	Umbilical cord

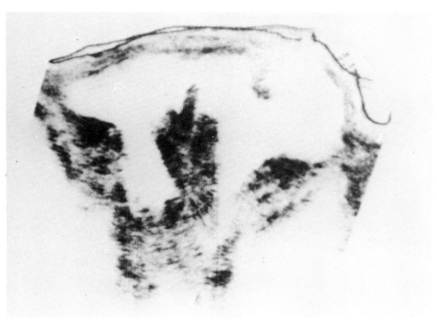

Fig. 113

Anencephaly; Hydrocephaly

An elevated alpha fetoprotein in the amniotic fluid very often indicates a neural tube defect. One of the commoner reasons for elevation of the alpha fetoprotein is anencephaly. Figures 114 and 115 are examples of an ultrasound examination on anencephalic fetuses. It is extremely important to attempt to line up the fetal body with the supposed site of the fetal head when trying to detect an anencephalic fetus. If the fetal body can be lined up correctly, a cluster of echoes can be visualized in the region of the fetal head. This cluster of echoes is fairly characteristic for an anencephalic fetus.

Figure 114 demonstrates numerous ill-defined echoes in the region of the fetal head. These are not the characteristic echoes of a biparietal diameter. The discrepancy in size between the fetal head and the fetal body is noted. This is usually present in an anencephalic. Figure 115 is another example with a cluster of echoes in the region of the fetal head. Again, the diameter and size of the fetal head is smaller than expected for the size of the fetal body.

Figures 116 and 117 are examples of a hydrocephalic fetus. In this instance, the opposite size discrepancy is true. The head size is much larger than expected for the fetal body. In figure 116 the head is one-and-a-half times as large as expected for the size of the fetal body. In figure 117 the head size is not only large, but fairly sonolucent for its size. Hydrocephalus often is most easily diagnosed by real-time examination. In real-time studies the ventricles stand out more easily than on a B-scan examination.

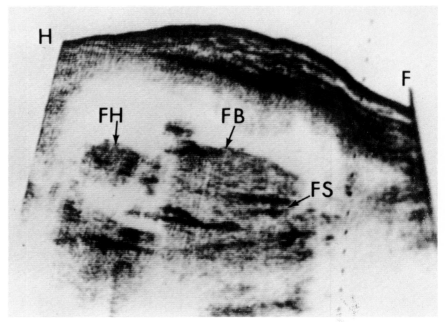

Fig. 114

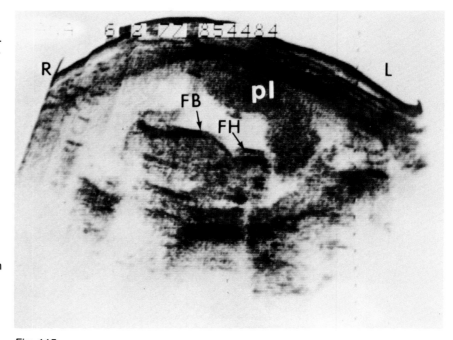

Fig. 115

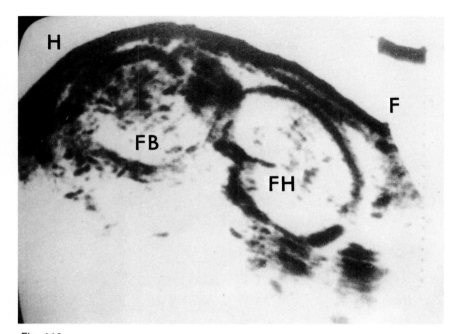

Fig. 116

SOURCE: Figures 116 and 117 are provided through the courtesy of Dr. M. Shaub, Centinela Valley Hospital, Los Angeles, California.

B	= Urinary bladder
F	= Foot
FB	= Fetal body
FH	= Fetal head
FS	= Fetal spine
H	= Head
L	= Left
Pl	= Placenta
R	= Right

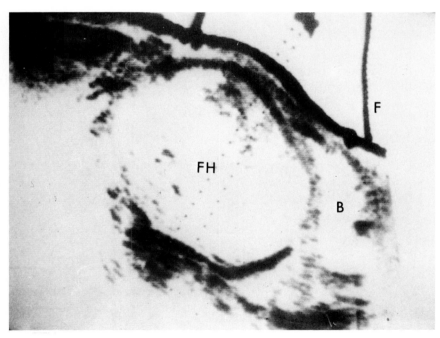

Fig. 117

Dandy-Walker Syndrome; Single Ventricle; IUGR; Triploidy

When examining the fetus during the course of an obstetrical study, we may find a discrepancy between the size of the fetal head and body. It then becomes necessary to determine whether or not the head, the body, or one of the two is inordinately "small for dates." In this instance, it is important to have an adequate menstrual history in an effort to determine the abnormality. Figure 118 is a scan of a fetus with a markedly enlarged fetal head. There are no echoes noted within the head, indicating that it is a fluid-filled structure. The size of the head is markedly enlarged compared with the size of the fetal body. This was an extremely unusual case of an abnormally dilated fourth ventricle in the Dandy-Walker syndrome. Not only is the head size abnormal, but its sonolucent appearance indicates that the abnormality is in the head and not in the fetal body.

Figure 119 is another example of a markedly enlarged and sonolucent head in comparison to the fetal body. As in figure 118, the fetal head is relatively sonolucent, indicating that it is a fluid-filled structure. This case turned out to be a single ventricle in which the brain substance was markedly compressed, secondary to the ventricular fluid.

Occasionally, however, we encounter a fetus in which the fetal body is actually small compared to a normally sized head. One of the more common reasons for this is intrauterine-growth retardation. Often, the fetus will spare the fetal brain at the expense of the fetal body in the entity of intrauterine growth retardation.

Figure 120 is an example of such a case. There is a normally sized fetal head and an abnormally small fetal body. This actually represents fetal wasting, secondary to growth retardation. Total intrauterine volume has been used to diagnose intrauterine-growth retardation earlier than has been previously possible. This severe degree of growth retardation, with the fetal body smaller than the fetal head, usually is an ominous sign.

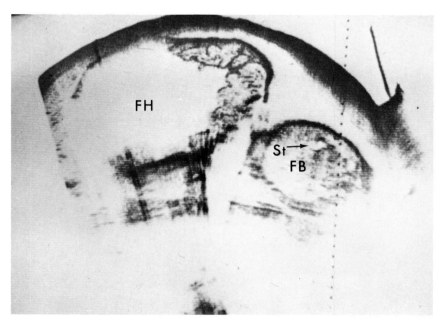

Fig. 118

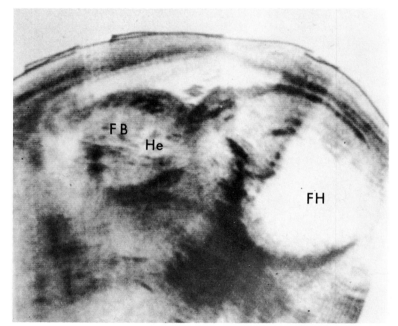

Fig. 119

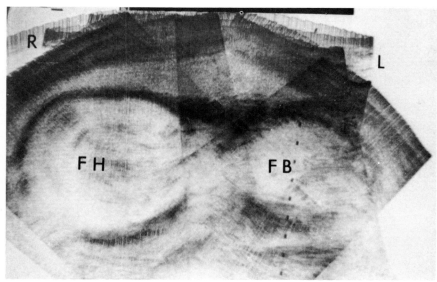

Fig. 120

Figure 121 is a case of an abnormally small fetal body in early pregnancy at approximately 20 weeks. In this instance, the fetal head was of normal size and growing at a normal rate. The fetal body, however, not only was abnormally small, but its growth rate was decreased over the normal range. Because of the ultrasonic findings, the patient underwent an elective abortion. She was found to have a triploidy (69 chromosomes) in which the fetal head was within normal size, and the fetal body was abnormally small.

SOURCE: The case for figure 119 is provided through the courtesy of Dr. R. Filly, University of California, San Francisco, California.

FB = Fetal body
FC = Falx cerebri
FH = Fetal head
FS = Fetal spine
He = Heart
L = Left
R = Right
St = Stomach

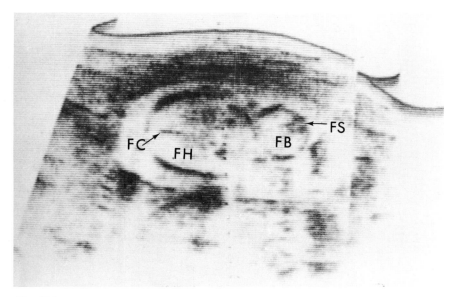

Fig. 121

Cystic Lymphangioma

During the course of an ultrasound examination, an inordinate amount of fluid may be found and the diagnosis of polyhydramnios made. We should, however, look closely at the fluid to make sure that is free within the uterine cavity. Very rarely, a fluid-filled mass contained within a curvilinear echo will be seen.

Figures 122–125 represent two separate cases with large fluid-filled masses contained within a structure that appears to be attached to the fetus. The possibility of a meningocele or meningo-myelocele was strongly considered. Both of these cases are examples of cystic lymphangiomas arising from the fetal neck and base of the skull. Figures 122 and 123 show the large fluid-filled mass contained within a structure which appears to be separate from the amniotic fluid. In figure 123, the mass is situated in close proximity to the fetal head.

Figures 124 and 125 are another case, again with a large sonolucent mass. Figure 125 is the more important scan in that the curvilinear echo demonstrates that the fluid-filled mass is not amniotic fluid. If it were secondary to amniotic fluid, the fetus would be seen floating more freely in the uterine cavity. In most of these cases, the fetus is situated on one side of the uterine cavity, because it is displaced by the large cystic mass.

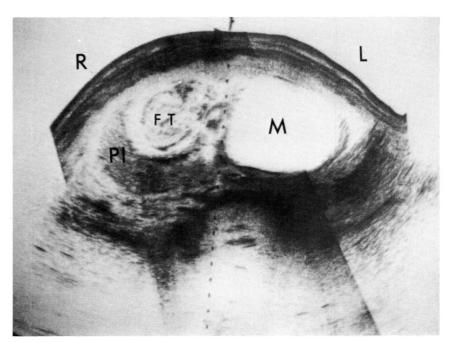

Fig. 122

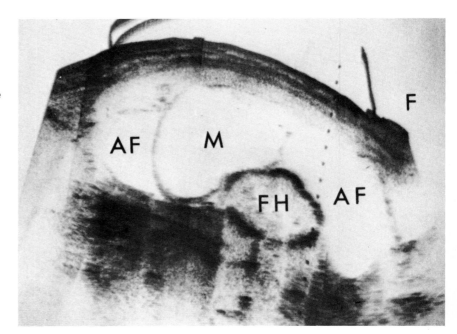

Fig. 123

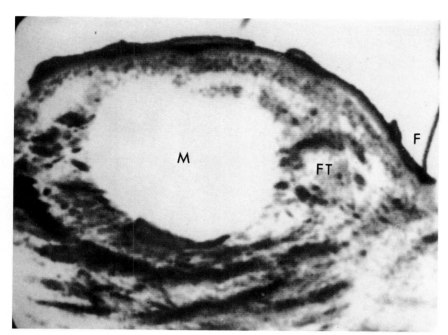

Fig. 124

Source: Figures 124 and 125 are provided through the courtesy of Dr. M. Shaub, Centinela Valley Hospital, Los Angeles, California.

AF	=	Amniotic fluid
F	=	Foot
FH	=	Fetal head
FT	=	Fetal trunk
L	=	Left
M	=	Cystic lymphangioma
Pl	=	Placenta
R	=	Right

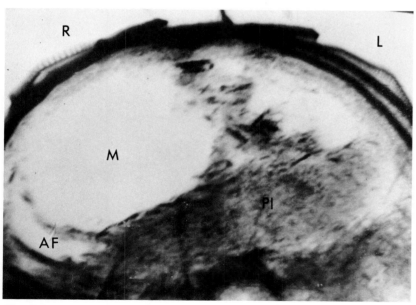

Fig. 125

Jejunal Atresia; Prune-belly Syndrome; Omphalocele

We normally can see fluid in the fetal stomach during a fetal examination. The urinary bladder of the fetus may also be fluid-filled. Very rarely, a few small lucencies in the abdomen will be noted secondary to normal filling of the small bowel with amniotic fluid. If there is an inordinate amount of bowel loops or sonolucent masses present in the abdomen, it is necessary to scrutinize the fetus in closer detail. Figure 126 demonstrates numerous sonolucent structures which remained fairly well fixed in position in the fetal abdomen during the course of an ultrasound examination. Three large sonolucent circular structures, which represent fluid-filled bowel, are seen. This fetus was eventually diagnosed as having jejeunal atresia. Very often, a high gastrointestinal obstruction in the fetus can lead to polyhydramnios. When fluid-filled structures within the fetus, which do not change position, are seen the possibility of a gastrointestional obstruction should be considered.

Figures 127 and 128 are another example of a fetus with numerous large circular and tubular fluid-filled structures. In this instance, however, the fluid-filled structures were secondary to the genitourinary tract. This was found to be hydroureter and hydronephrosis, secondary to prune-belly syndrome. We see the large fluid-filled ureters filling the entire abdomen and causing marked distention of the fetal abdomen. Because of the large abdomen, a cesarean section had to be performed in order to deliver the fetus.

Figure 129 is an unusual case with the fetal abdominal contents visualized outside the fetal body. This is a case of an omphalocele. Fetal omphalocele will elevate the alpha fetal proteins as will neural tube defects. When examining a fetus with an elevated alpha fetal protein, not only should the cervical and sacral regions be studied for meningoceles, but also the anterior abdomen should be inspected to rule out an omphalocele.

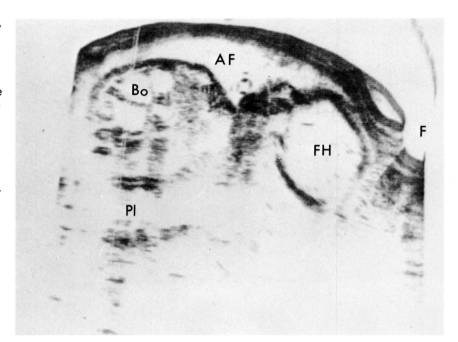

Fig. 126

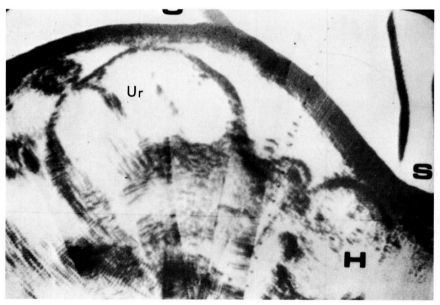

Fig. 127

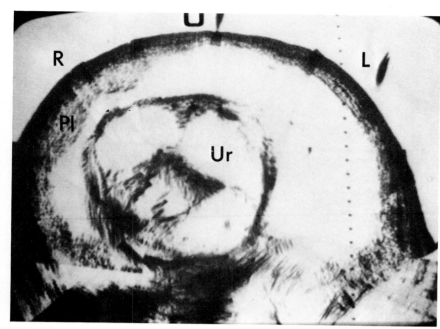

Fig. 128

SOURCE: Figure 126 is provided through the courtesy of Dr. R. Hoffman, Torrance Memorial Hospital, Torrance, California.

Figure 129 is provided through the courtesy of Dr. D. McQuown, Long Beach Memorial Hospital, Long Beach, California.

Ab	=	Abdominal contents outside the fetal body secondary to an omphalocele
AF	=	Amniotic fluid
Bo	=	Dilated bowel secondary to jejeunal atresia
F	=	Foot
FB	=	Fetal body
FH	=	Fetal head
H	=	Fetal head
L	=	Left
Pl	=	Placenta
S	=	Level of the symphysis pubis
R	=	Right
U	=	Level of the umbilicus
Ur	=	Dilated ureter secondary to prune-belly

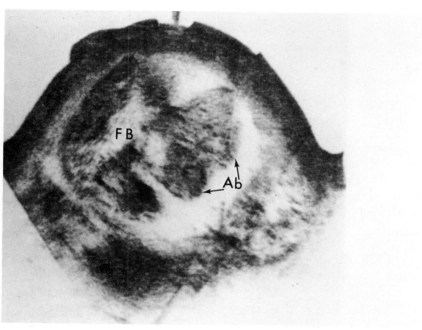

Fig. 129

Fetal Ascites

Fetal ascites presents ultrasonic findings similar to those seen in the adult. Fetal ascites can occur in a patient with Rh sensitization. When the fetus is severely affected with Rh incompatibility, marked ascites can develop. Figure 130 is a longitudinal scan of the fetus with a large amount of ascitic fluid. The abdomen is somewhat enlarged, secondary to the amount of ascitic fluid. Cephalad to the ascitic fluid, the highly echogenic liver is seen. Figure 131 is a transverse scan of the upper abdomen with the characteristic findings of ascites similar to that found in the adult. The ascitic fluid is situated between the abdominal wall and the liver, which is floating away from the abdominal wall. The circular structure in the liver is secondary to a dilated umbilical vein. Figure 132 is an interesting transverse scan of the fetus. The umbilical cord, as it enters the fetal abdomen, actually can be seen. It divides in the ascitic fluid as it enters the fetal abdomen.

Ultrasound can be used to assist in fetal transfusions. Used in conjunction with fluoroscopy, the fluoroscopy time can be decreased markedly. Figure 133 is a scan performed on the lateral aspect of the mother while a fetal transfusion was being performed. Here we see the needle as it enters the fetal abdomen. It is easily detected because of the surrounding ascitic fluid.

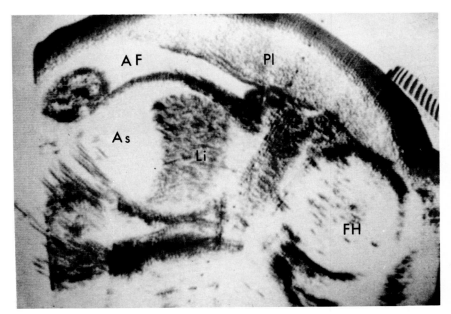

Fig. 130

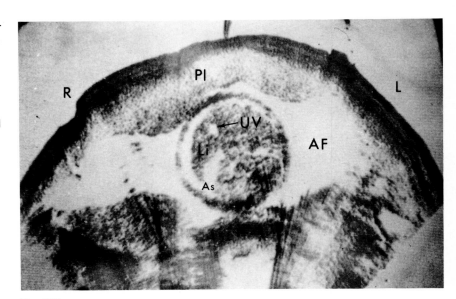

Fig. 131

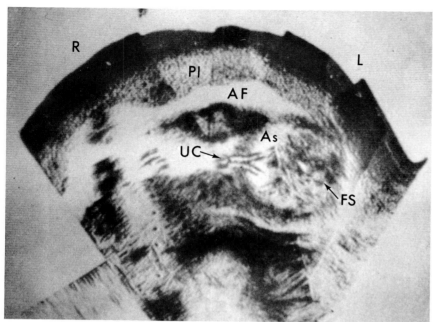

AF	=	Amniotic fluid
As	=	Ascitic fluid
FH	=	Fetal head
FS	=	Fetal spine
L	=	Left
Li	=	Liver
N	=	Transfusion needle
Pl	=	Placenta
R	=	Right
UC	=	Umbilical cord
UV	=	Umbilical vein

Fig. 132

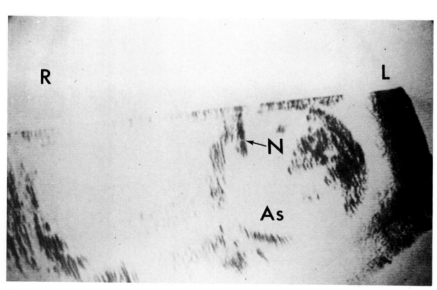

Fig. 133

Maternal Anatomy

Often, when scanning the pregnant uterus, sonolucent structures are visualized posterior to the uterus. Very often, this represents the maternal aorta and inferior vena cava if it is near the midline. We will, however, occasionally see a sonolucent structure posterior to the lateral aspect of the uterus. Figure 134 is a transverse scan with a circular structure posterior to the uterus on the right side. This represents a dilated right ureter. Of course, this is a common finding in pregnancy, since right hydroureter and hydronephrosis is often seen. Figure 135 is a longitudinal scan which attempts to delineate further the right ureter. The dilated tubular ureter is seen on top of the right iliopsoas muscle. The placenta and amniotic fluid are anterior to the right ureter.

Figure 136 is a longitudinal scan of the right kidney in the supine position. There is evidence of mild hydronephrosis secondary to the right hydroureter. Occasionally, when examining the lower uterine segment, a sonolucent structure is seen posterior to the vagina. Figure 137 is an example of such a case; fluid is actually seen in the rectum. This may be seen following enemas or in cases where the mother is suffering from gastrointestinal problems.

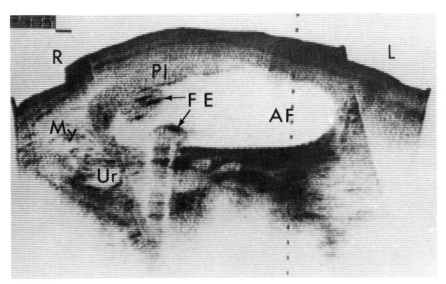

Fig. 134

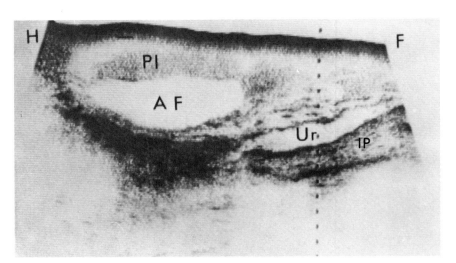

Fig. 135

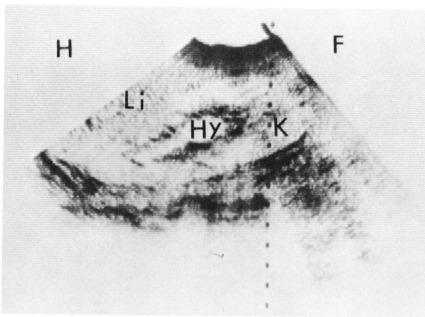

AF	=	Amniotic fluid
B	=	Urinary bladder
F	=	Foot
FE	=	Fetal extremities
GS	=	Gestational sac
H	=	Head
Hy	=	Mild hydronephrosis
IP	=	Iliopsoas muscle
K	=	Kidney
L	=	Left
Li	=	Liver
My	=	Myometrium
Pl	=	Placenta
R	=	Right
Re	=	Fluid-filled rectum
Ur	=	Dilated right ureter
V	=	Vagina

Fig. 136

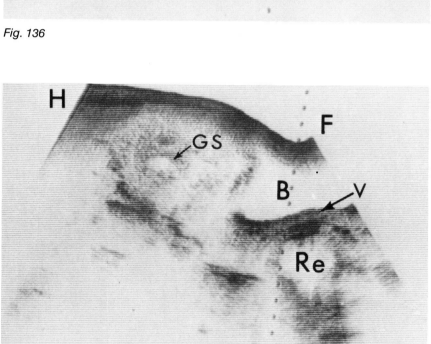

Fig. 137

Fetal Death   I.

If there is any question as to fetal viability, it is important to do a Doppler or real-
time examination in an effort to detect
fetal cardiac activity. Several signs,
however, give evidence of fetal death on
a routine B-scan examination. The most
common sign is finding fetal edema
about the head or the body. Although
this is not automatically consistent with
fetal death, it is highly suspicious. Fetal
edema and congestive heart failure may
be seen in the fetus. Figures 138
and 139 are examples of fetal edema
registering as a double ring sign around
the fetal head. Edema is usually seen
entirely around the fetal head. Mistakes
can be made when the fetus is in close
contact to the urinary bladder which will
give a false double ring sign.

Another sign of fetal death is evidence
of collapse of the normal contour of the
fetal head. Figure 140 is an example
of distortion of the fetal head. Marked
straightening (arrows) of the fetal contour which is markedly abnormal is
noted. When we see abnormality of the
fetal skull, a Doppler or real-time examination should be performed. Figure
141 is an example of the overlapping
of the skull bones which is another sign
of fetal death. Ultrasonic visualization
of overlapping of the fetal skull has the
same significance as the X-ray finding
of an overlapping skull. Both suggest
fetal death.

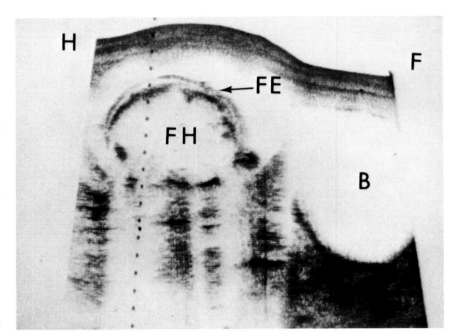

Fig. 138

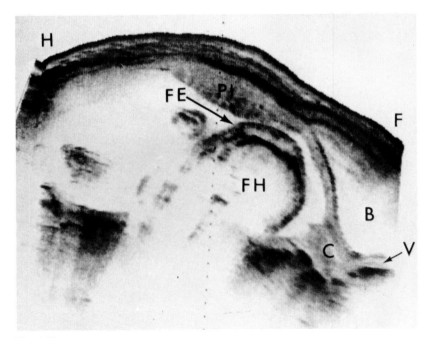

Fig. 139

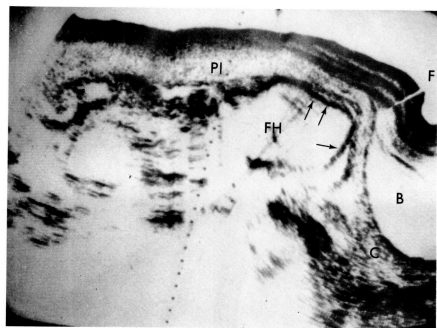

Arrows	=	Distortion of fetal skull (fig. 140)
Arrows	=	Overlapping skull echoes (fig. 141)
B	=	Urinary bladder
C	=	Cervix
F	=	Foot
FC	=	Falx cerebri
FE	=	Fetal edema
FH	=	Fetal head
H	=	Head
PI	=	Placenta
V	=	Vagina

Fig. 140

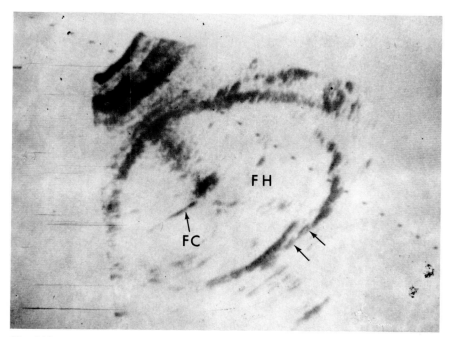

Fig. 141

Fetal Death   II.

Another indication of fetal death is the empty fetal thorax sign. When the fetal thorax is markedly distorted, this should be considered. Figures 142 and 143 are of a twin pregnancy. One of the twins is no longer viable. Here we see the empty-thorax sign. The normal echo pattern of the fetal thorax is not seen. Instead, the thorax appears more lucent with coarser echoes within it. There is a marked distortion of the contour of the fetal thorax compared with normal fetal body seen in figure 143. The normal circular-to-oval structure of the fetal thorax is lost. We are seeing evidence of degeneration of the fetus with collapse of the fetal thorax, similar to collapse of the fetal skull.

Figure 144 is an example of distortion of the fetal spine (arrows). Normally the fetal spine is fairly straight on longitudinal scan. Marked distortion and angulation of the fetal spine, however, are present. This ultrasonic finding corresponds to the marked angulation in fetal death on X-ray. We again see evidence of fetal degeneration when this marked anatomic distortion takes place. Figure 145 is an example of collapse of the fetal head and the fetal body. We see severe oligohydramnios along with marked difficulty in visualizing the normal fetal structures.

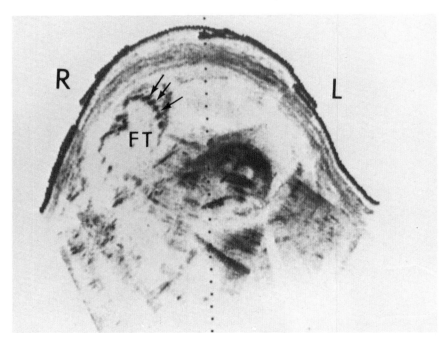

Fig. 142

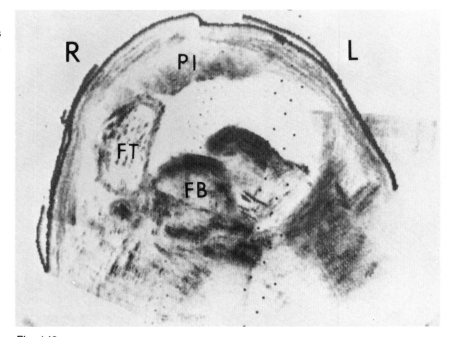

Fig. 143

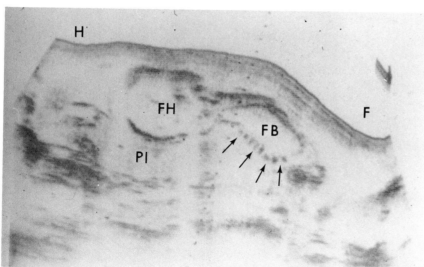

Fig. 144

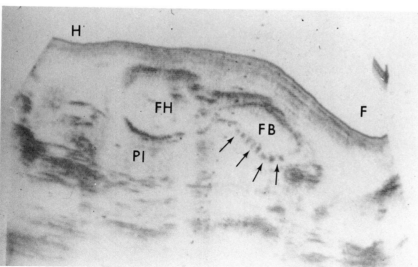

Fig. 145

Fetal Death   III.

Separation of the amnion from the chorion may be visualized in fetal death. During early pregnancy, the amnion and chorion are not in contact. Chorionic fluid is found between the amnion and chorion. By approximately the eighteenth to twentieth week of pregnancy, the amnion and chorion come into contact, with no evidence of any space between them. In some instances of fetal demise, however, fluid may collect between the amnion and chorion, separating the amnion from the placenta and the surrounding uterine cavity. The case in figures 146–149 is an example of separation of the amnion (arrows) from the chorion. The potential space of the chorionic cavity is now filled with fluid. Sometimes, this finding can be mistaken for a fetal abnormality such as a meningomyelocele or other fluid collection attached to the fetus. When examining the fetus closely, however, we often find that this curvilinear echo is completely surrounding the fetus. It actually represents separation of the amnionic membrane from the lining of the uterine cavity.

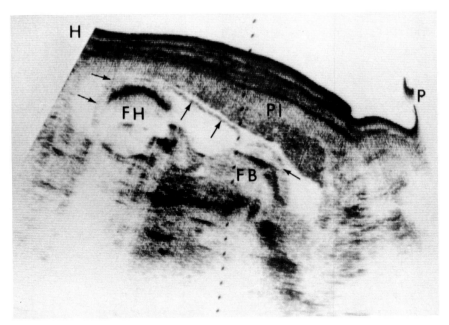

Fig. 146

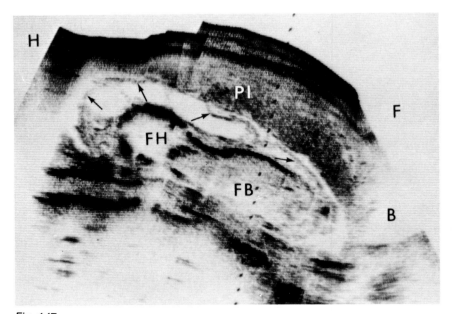

Fig. 147

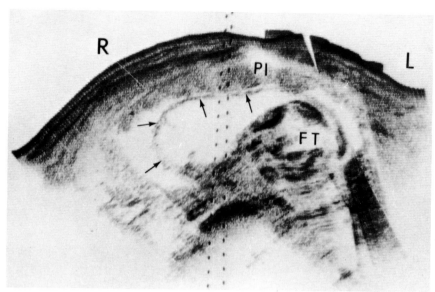

Fig. 148

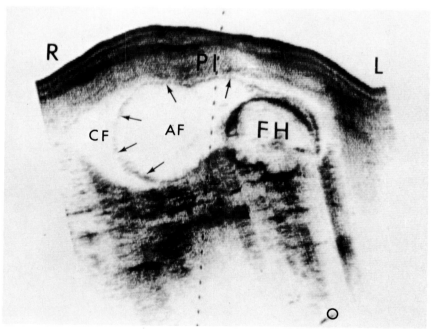

Fig. 149

Arrows	=	Amnionic membrane
AF	=	Amniotic fluid
B	=	Urinary bladder
CF	=	Chorionic fluid
F	=	Foot
FB	=	Fetal body
FH	=	Fetal head
FT	=	Fetal thorax
H	=	Head
L	=	Left
P	=	Level of the symphysis pubis
PI	=	Placenta
R	=	Right

Incompetent Cervix   I.

The incompetent cervix is clinically described as a painless, bloodless, dilation of the endocervical canal, usually occurring during the second trimester of pregnancy. Ultrasound can easily visualize fluid in the endocervical canal and therefore confirm the diagnosis of incompetent cervix. Figure 150 is a longitudinal examination demonstrating the normal appearance of the endocervical canal. The endocervical canal appears as a strong linear echo in the mid portion of the myometrial echoes of the cervix. The normal length of the endocervical canal varies from approximately 2.5–6 cm. There should be no evidence of fluid in the endocervical canal during the course of a normal pregnancy. When examining a patient for incompetent cervix, it is important to have the bladder well filled. Overdistention of the bladder, however, may actually lead to collapse of an incompetent cervix.

Figure 151 is an example of a longitudinal scan in a patient with incompetent cervix and an overdistended bladder. The urinary bladder is markedly distended and actually compressing the cervix. The patient was asked to partially void to relieve bladder pressure. Figure 152 is a scan of the same patient following partial bladder emptying. Now the fluid in the endocervical canal confirms the diagnosis of an incompetent cervix.

We now routinely examine a patient suspected of having an incompetent cervix with a full urinary bladder and partial bladder emptying. If the bladder is markedly overdistended, it may cause closure of an incompetent cervix. Figure 153 is a transverse scan through an incompetent cervix with fluid in the endocervical canal.

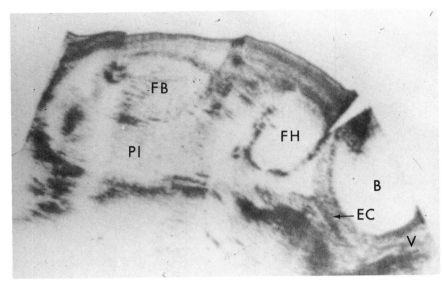

Fig. 150

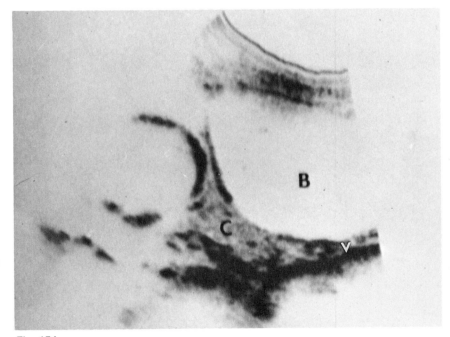

Fig. 151

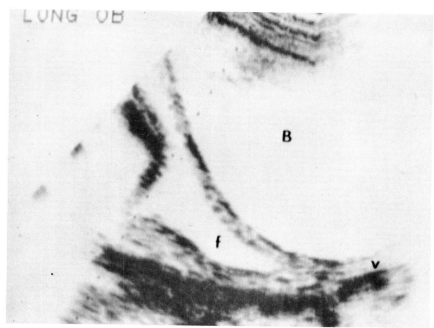

B   = Urinary bladder
C   = Cervix
EC = Normal endocervical canal
f   = Fluid in the endocervical canal, sec-
      ondary to incompetent cervix
FB = Fetal body
FH = Fetal head
PI = Placenta
V   = Vagina
v   = Vagina

Fig. 152

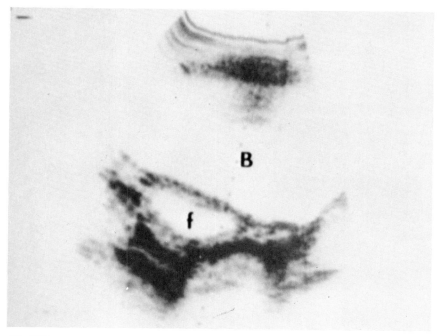

Fig. 153

Incompetent Cervix   II.

Figure 154 is another example of incompetent cervix with amniotic fluid in the endocervical canal. The amniotic fluid is visualized almost to the external os. When examining a patient for incompetent cervix, it is important to align the transducer parallel to the long axis of the endocervical canal. This is best determined on the transverse scans by marking the right and left border of the cervix on the patient's skin. Longitudinal scans are then begun parallel to the long axis of the cervix.

Figure 155 is an example of incompetent cervix in a twin pregnancy. A cephalic fetus with the fetal head near the internal os is seen. Amniotic fluid is noted in the endocervical canal, again nearly completely to the external os. A second fetus is noted in the breech position in the fundal region of the uterus.

Figures 156 and 157 are examples of another case of incompetent cervix. There is markedly severe dilation. of the endocervical canal by amniotic fluid. This patient had marked bulging membranes; this is easily visualized on the ultrasound examination. Amniotic fluid is seen actually bulging into the proximal vagina.

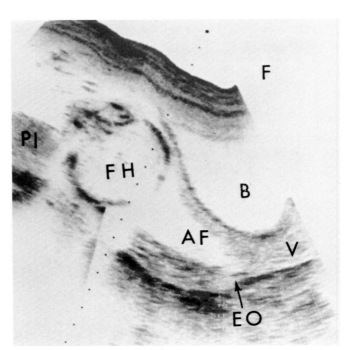

Fig. 154

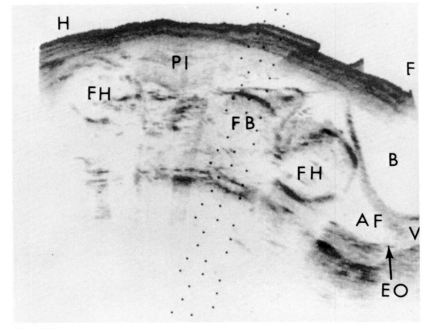

Fig. 155

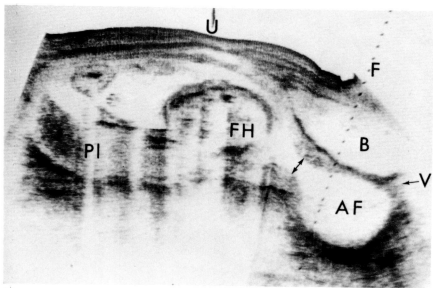

Fig. 156

AF = Amniotic fluid
B   = Urinary bladder
EO = External os
F   = Foot
FB = Fetal body
FH = Fetal head
H   = Head
L   = Left
PI = Placenta
R   = Right
U   = Umbilical level
V   = Vagina

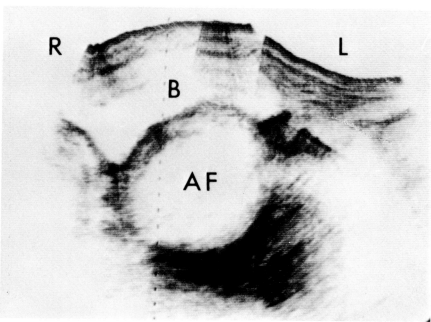

Fig. 157

Ectopic Pregnancy   I.

Patients are often sent for ultrasound examination to rule out ectopic pregnancy. Often, they have a positive pregnancy test and pelvic or lower abdominal pain. The ultrasound examination initially centers on visualizing the uterus to determine whether or not a gestational sac is present. If the uterus is empty the study then concentrates on visualizing the adnexal regions to determine whether or not a mass is present. Figure 158 is an example of an ectopic pregnancy with the gestational sac within the tube on the right side. Here we see strong surrounding echoes, indicating decidual reaction. Even some internal echoes arise from the fetus within the gestational sac in the right adnexa. Strong linear echoes are present in the uterus, secondary to a Lippe's loop as seen in figure 159. The intrauterine device has the characteristic steplike pattern of a Lippe's loop. Figure 160 is a longitudinal scan of the same patient with the gestational sac situated in the right tube. Most ectopic pregnancies are not quite this classic. If we see a classic gestational sac within the tube, the diagnosis is quite easy.

Figure 161 is another example of an ectopic pregnancy on the right side. Fetal echoes inside the fluid-filled gestational sac are seen. Also noted in the pelvis are areas of hemorrhage behind the uterus and right adnexa. This is a common occurrence with some pelvic fluid secondary to hemorrhage associated with the ectopic pregnancy.

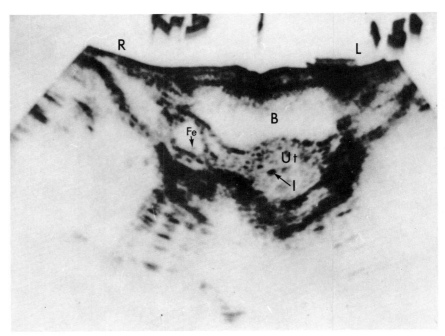

Fig. 158

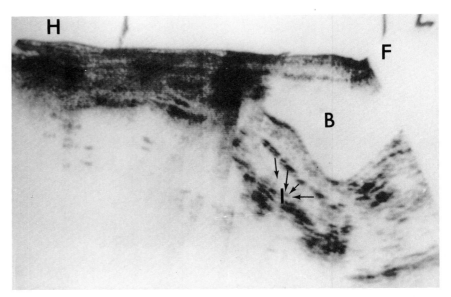

Fig. 159

SOURCE: The case in figures 158–160 is provided through the courtesy of Dr. M. Shaub, Centinela Valley Hospital, Los Angeles, California.

B	= Urinary bladder
F	= Foot
Fe	= Fetal echoes
GS	= Gestational sacs
H	= Head
He	= Hemorrhage
I and arrows	= Intrauterine device
L	= Left
R	= Right
Ut	= Uterus

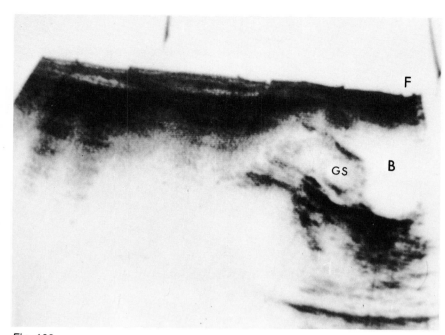

Fig. 160

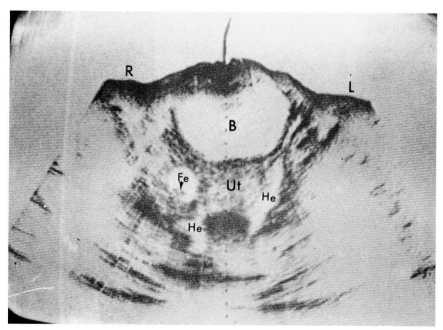

Fig. 161

Ectopic Pregnancy II.

The usual ultrasonic finding in ectopic pregnancy is an ill-defined adnexal mass rather than a clearly defined gestational sac, as noted previously. Figures 162 and 163 are scans of a patient with an ectopic pregnancy in the right adnexal region. The transverse scan in figure 162 demonstrates a solid-appearing echogenic mass that is larger than the normally sized left ovary. No gestational sac is clearly discernible. This is a more characteristic appearance of an ectopic pregnancy. A small central echo (arrow) is noted within the uterus. Often in an ectopic pregnancy, endometrial proliferation will be noted within the uterine cavity and may even have the appearance of a false gestational sac. This is the normal uterine response to the pregnant state, even though the pregnancy is outside the uterus.

The case in figures 164 and 165 is another characteristic ultrasonic appearance to an ectopic pregnancy. Figure 164 is a longitudinal scan of the right adnexal region with a mixed echogenic mass in the right adnexa. This fluid- and solid-containing mass was secondary to an ectopic pregnancy. Also noted in this patient was fluid situated in the cul-de-sac posterior to the uterus. This is seen in figure 165, and the fluid was secondary to hemorrhage from the ectopic pregnancy.

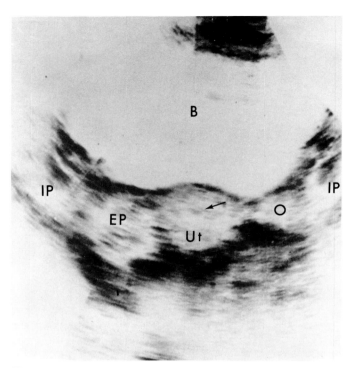

Fig. 162

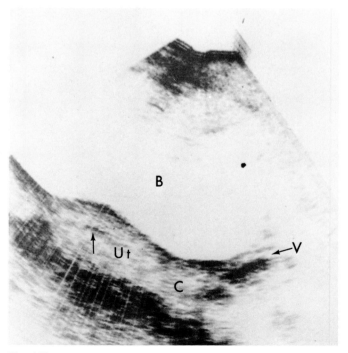

Fig. 163

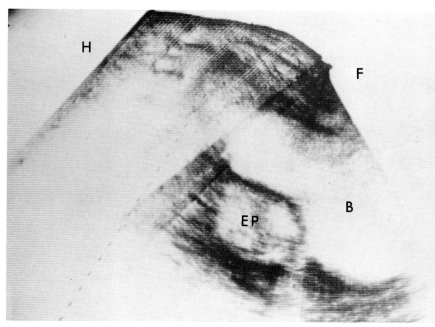

Arrow = Endometrial proliferation
B = Urinary bladder
C = Cervix
EP = Ectopic pregnancy
F = Foot
Fl = Fluid in the cul-de-sac
H = Head
IP = Iliopsoas muscles
O = Normal left ovary
Ut = Uterus
V = Vagina

Fig. 164

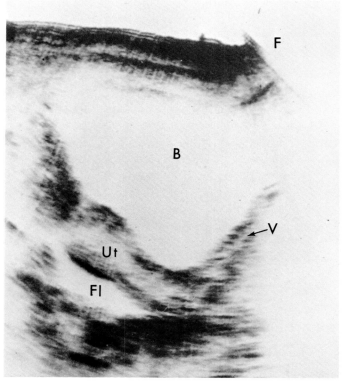

Fig. 165

Ectopic Pregnancy   III.

Frequently, an ectopic pregnancy yields a large ill-defined mass in the pelvis very adherent to the uterus. When the borders between the uterus and the mass are lost, the findings can be similar to chronic pelvic inflammatory disease or endometriosis. The case in figures 166–168 is such an instance in which a chronic ectopic pregnancy is quite similar to chronic pelvic inflammatory disease. In figure 166 the ectopic pregnancy is present on the right side with a gestational sac surrounded by echogenic material. It is difficult to distinguish the border between the chronic ectopic pregnancy and the uterus. Within the uterus is a central echo consistent with endometrial proliferation. Posterior to the uterus is fluid in the cul-de-sac. Figure 167 is a longitudinal scan in the midline, again with endometrial proliferation within the uterus. Posterior to the uterus is the fluid in the cul-de-sac. Scanning to the right side of the patient, we see the gestational sac in figure 168 on a longitudinal scan. The highly echogenic material surrounding the gestational sac, which is secondary to hemorrhage and debris, is visualized.

Occasionally, a chronic ectopic pregnancy can reach a fairly large size. Figure 169 is a longitudinal scan in the midline with a chronic ectopic pregnancy, which could be confused with a myomatous uterus. There is a loss of the tissue planes between the uterus and the chronic ectopic pregnancy, so that we cannot visualize the uterine borders.

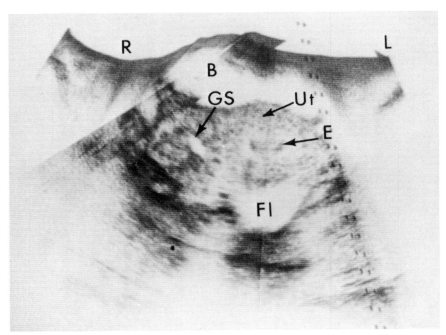

Fig. 166

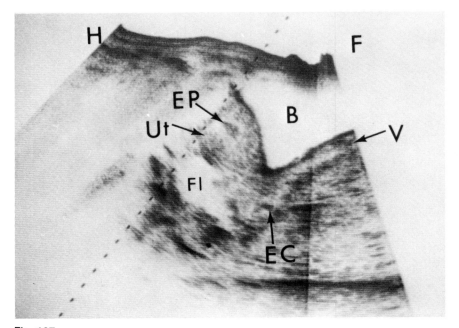

Fig. 167

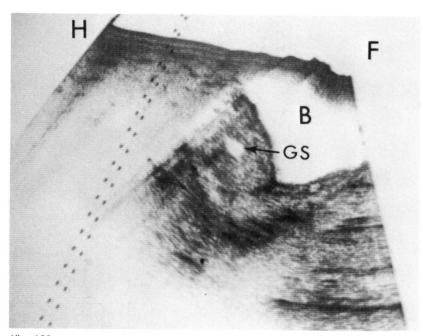

Fig. 168

SOURCE: Figure 169 is provided through the courtesy of Dr. M. Shaub, Centinela Valley Hospital, Los Angeles, California.

B	=	Urinary bladder
C	=	Chronic ectopic pregnancy
E	=	Endometrial cavity
EC	=	Endocervical canal
EP	=	Endometrial proliferation
F	=	Foot
Fl	=	Fluid in the cul-de-sac
GS	=	Gestational sac
H	=	Head
L	=	Left
M	=	Mass (ectopic pregnancy)
R	=	Right
Ut	=	Uterus
V	=	Vagina

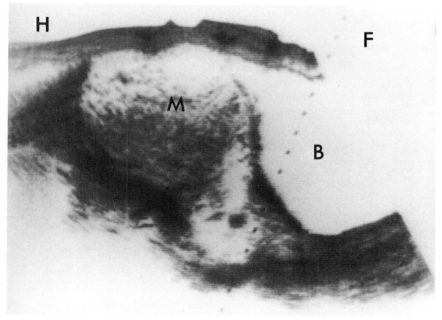

Fig. 169

Intrauterine Devices Associated with Pregnancy

Ultrasound examination is often requested to locate an intrauterine device. If this request occurs during the first 10 weeks of pregnancy, the exam can be successful. During this time period, the intrauterine device will stand out as a strong echo adjacent to the gestational sac. If it is after the tenth or eleventh week of pregnancy, however, numerous fetal echoes are present within the uterine cavity. The strong echoes arising from the fetus will make distinguishing the fetus from the intrauterine device difficult.

The gestational sac is seen as a fluid-filled structure in the mid portion of the uterus in figure 170. A strong circular echo is noted in the myometrium on the right side of the uterus. This is secondary to a Copper 7 intrauterine device. Figure 171 is a longitudinal scan through the mid portion of the uterus, demonstrating the gestational sac with fetal echoes within it. Figure 172 is the same patient; the right side of the uterus is being scanned. The strong echo of the intrauterine device is seen. The intrauterine device can be visualized at this time in the pregnancy, because the echoes arising from the fetus are not numerous enough to give any difficulty. Figure 173 is another example of a gestational sac present in conjunction with an intrauterine device. Here we see the gestational sac on the right side of the uterus. The strong circular echo is the characteristic echo arising from a Copper 7 intrauterine device on the left half of the uterus.

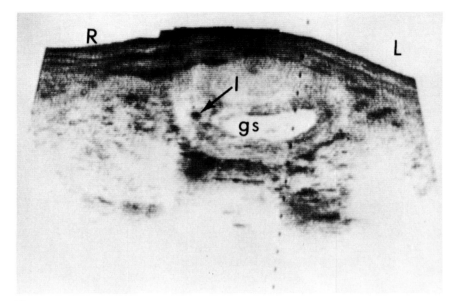

Fig. 170

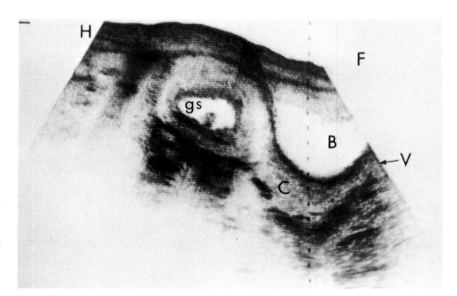

Fig. 171

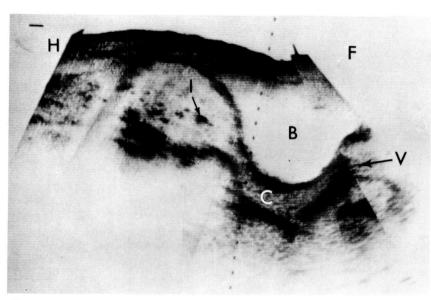

B	= Urinary bladder
C	= Cervix
F	= Foot
gs	= Gestational sac
H	= Head
I	= Intrauterine device
L	= Left
R	= Right
V	= Vagina

Fig. 172

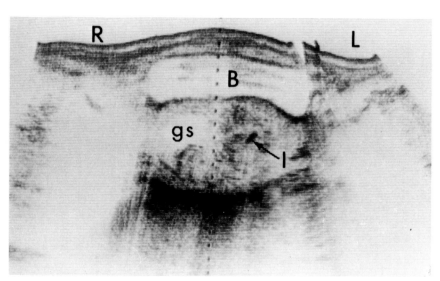

Fig. 173

Bicornuate Uterus

Occasionally, we will encounter a pregnancy in a bicornuate uterus, with a gestational sac on one side and myometrial
echoes on the other side. The case
in figures 174–176 is from a patient who requested a therapeutic abortion. Following a D and C, no gestational
products were removed. Consequently,
the patient underwent ultrasound examination. Figure 174 is a transverse
scan following the attempted therapeutic abortion. We find evidence of a
gestational sac with fetal echoes on the
right side of the uterus. On the left side
of the uterus there is a mixed echo pattern consistent with hemorrhage.
Myometrium is present between the
gestational sac and hemorrhage. Because of this finding, the diagnosis of a
bicornuate uterus was made. We then
lined up the gestational sac with the
cervix and obtained an oblique longitudinal scan in figure 175. Here we see
the pregnant cornua with a gestational
sac in the fundal region of the uterus. A
second oblique longitudinal scan was
obtained, lining up the area of hemorrhage with the cervix. This is shown in
figure 176. The other cornua with
hemorrhage is visualized and lined up
with the cervix and vagina. This is evidence of a pregnancy in a bicornuate
uterus. The therapeutic abortion was not
successful because the nonpregnant
cornua was entered.

Figure 177 is another example of a
pregnancy in a bicornate uterus. The
gestational sac is seen on the right side.
In the left cornua we see strong high-
amplitude echoes, indicating endometrial proliferation in the nonpregnant
cornua.

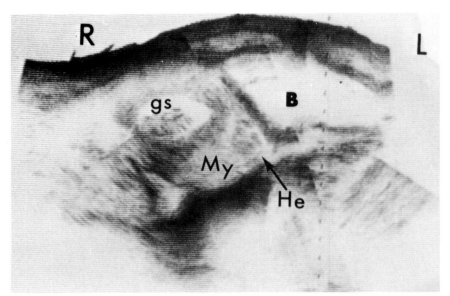

Fig. 174

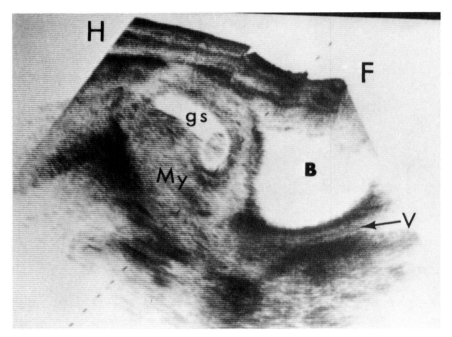

Fig. 175

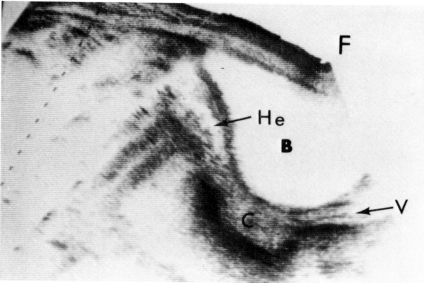

B   = Urinary bladder
C   = Cervix
EP = Endometrial proliferation
F   = Foot
GS = Gestational sac
gs = Gestational sac
H   = Head
He = Hemorrhage
L   = Left
My = Myometrium
R   = Right
V   = Vagina

Fig. 176

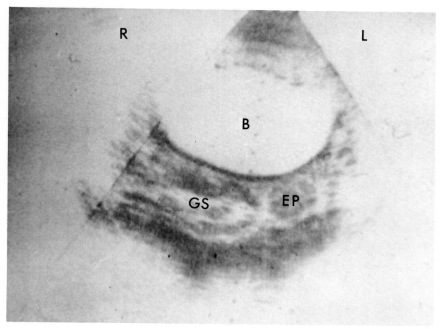

Fig. 177

Gynecologic Application of Ultrasound

Ultrasound of the pelvis is helpful to the referring physician trying to (1) confirm the presence of a pelvic mass, (2) describe the site of origin of a pelvic mass, (3) characterize the nature of such masses, (4) evaluate the pelvis of a patient who is difficult to examine clinically, and (5) detect fluid in the pelvis. Many pathologic entities in the pelvis have a similar ultrasound appearance; however, a combination of clinical history and ultrasound findings narrows the differential and usually leads to the correct diagnosis.

Technique

Certain difficulties are inherent in pelvic ultrasonography because of the location in the body. The pelvic organs are surrounded by numerous bony structures and air-filled bowel loops that are not penetrated by ultrasound. Measures must be taken to work around these technical limitations.

Production of an adequate pelvic scan requires that the patient have a distended urinary bladder. The patient is instructed to drink several glasses of water approximately 45 minutes prior to the examination. A urine-distended bladder stretches and elevates the pelvic organs, lifting small bowel loops out of the pelvis and providing an ultrasonic window for visualization of the pelvic organs. It often is necessary that the urinary bladder is distended to a degree that the patient is exceedingly uncomfortable. Some patients may not be able to tolerate a level of bladder filling necessary for adequate visualization. In such instances, the urinary bladder may be filled via a catheter, although this usually is unnecessary.

A 3.5-MHz transducer most commonly is used with 5.0-or 2.25-MHz transducers used in specific situations. Either B-scan or real-time examinations are performed, depending upon available equipment. Linear array real-time scanning is difficult to perform in the pelvic area because of anatomy. A longitudinal scan with a linear array (large transducer) is hampered by the symphysis pubis. Sector real time or B-scanners are better able to visualize the lower uterine segment and vaginal region. These transducers can angle in a caudad direction near the symphysis pubis, whereas a large linear array transducer cannot.

Patients usually are supine for pelvic scans. Occasionally they should be positioned right posterior oblique or left posterior oblique depending upon the area to be studied. Because of the bony pelvis, prone scans are of no value. Transverse scans of the pelvis are often performed perpendicular to the patient's skin. Best visualization of anatomy is obtained when scans are performed perpendicular to the long axis of the uterus. This scanning plane tends to provide the best visual separation of the uterus and ovaries. In order to visualize the lower uterine segment and vaginal area on transverse scans, it is necessary to use a caudad angle. Although usually midline in position, the uterus may be deviated to the right or left. Transverse scans will demonstrate the position of the uterus and assist in determining the best axis for longitudinal scans. Longitudinal scans are obtained parallel to the long axis of the uterus.

The ovaries are best visualized on transverse and longitudinal scans by angling the transducer posterior and lateral. This usually will place the ovaries anterior to the internal iliac vessels, which are used as anatomic landmarks.

The degree of bladder filling plays an important role in the quality and interpretation of pelvic scans. If the bladder is not adequately distended, masses cephalad to the urinary bladder may be obscured by air-filled bowel loops. The degree of bladder filling has a direct effect on the parenchymal echo pattern of the uterus. The fundal portion of the uterus often is less echogenic than the mid and lower uterine segments because of the shape of the urinary bladder and the through-transmission phenomenon. Because the bladder is fluid filled, through transmission is greater over the wider region of the bladder. Since the lower uterine and cervical segments are posterior to this wider region, higher level parenchymal uterine echoes are visualized in these areas than in the fundal area.

Fluid-filled bowel loops present diagnostic difficulties during pelvic ultrasound examination. In order to fill the bladder adequately, the patient is required to drink a large quantity of water prior to the examination. This may cause numerous loops of small intestine to appear as fluid-filled masses posterior and cephalad to the urinary bladder. Misinterpretation of these normal structures for various pathologic processes may result. Such errors can be avoided by real-time examination or repeat studies. Real-time exams demonstrate peristaltic activity in fluid-filled bowel loops. A repeat examination will show a change or disappearance of the previously noted masses if they were secondary to fluid-filled bowel.

Stool in the rectosigmoid region may appear as a solid mass in the pelvis. This error can be avoided by a repeat study following laxative administration or by a water enema during real-time examination.

Normal Anatomy

The urinary bladder is echo free with sharp borders when it is distended with urine. Some echoes secondary to reverberation artifact are seen in the anterior portion (see Appendix). Since the urinary bladder is fluid filled, it is used as a standard in the pelvis to determine whether a mass is cystic. On transverse scans, the urinary bladder will have a rectangular to triangular appearance. On longitudinal scans, its shape will vary depending upon the degree of filling. The pelvic organs normally will slightly indent the contour of the urinary bladder. Evaluation of bladder contour is important in detecting pelvic tumors. An unusual indentation of the urinary bladder may be the first clue to the presence of a pelvic mass. An echogenic mass such as a dermoid may be lost in the high-amplitude surrounding pelvic echoes. Dermoid indentation on the bladder may be the only sign suggesting the presence of a mass. Fluid-filled or stool-filled bowel may also indent the urinary bladder. Once a contour deformity of the bladder is noted, close scrutiny of the area usually will determine whether it is secondary to a normal anatomic structure or a pathologic process.

The approximate size of the uterus in a normal adult female is $8 \times 4 \times 4$ cm. It will be smaller in the postmenopausal and larger in the multiparous patient. The uterus has a characteristic pear-shaped appearance on longitudinal scans parallel to its long axis and an oval shape on transverse scans perpendicular to its long axis. The parenchymal echoes of the uterus are fairly homogeneous, with variation occurring secondary to differences in urinary bladder thickness. Because of enhanced through transmission those portions of uterus posterior to the wider parts of the urinary bladder will have higher amplitude echoes than those deep to a narrower portion. High amplitude, linear echoes are present in the uterine cavity just prior and during menstruation. A linear echo arising from the endocervical canal also can be identified. The uterus normally indents the urinary bladder, especially if it is anteverted. Uterine position is best determined on longitudinal scans. A retroverted, retroflexed uterus is the most difficult to evaluate. In these instances, optimum studies necessitate a markedly distended urinary bladder almost to the point of patient discomfort. A retroverted, retroflexed uterus often is falsely diagnosed as myomatous if the urinary bladder is not adequately distended.

In order to visualize the vaginal region, caudad angulation on both longitudinal and transverse scans is necessary. The vagina has a characteristic ultrasound appearance of three parallel lines. Occasionally the urethra can be visualized coursing through the posterior, inferior bladder wall.

When evaluating the ovaries, the muscles of the pelvic side walls should be identified (Sample 1977; Sample, Lippe, and Gyepes 1977). The obturator internus, piriformis, and iliopsoas muscles have a typical appearance and location. It is necessary to recognize these structures so they will not be mistaken for the ovaries or pelvic masses.

The ovaries of normal, adult premenopausal women usually are visualized on pelvic ultrasound (Sample 1977; Zemlyn 1974). The approximate size of the ovaries is $3.5 \times 2.0 \times 2.0$ cm, but this is variable. Occasionally one dimension of the ovary may appear larger because the distal end of the fallopian tube is included in the scan. The echo amplitude of the ovaries is slightly less than that of the uterus. The ovaries usually are situated in the adnexal regions lateral to the uterus. In order to visualize these regions, transverse and longitudinal scans must be angled posteriorly and laterally. When performed correctly, the internal iliac vessels and ureters can be seen deep to the ovaries. These anatomic landmarks are helpful in localizing the ovaries. The ovaries, however, may not be in the expected location lateral to the uterus. The cul-de-sac, superior to the uterine fundus, and anterior to the upper uterus are other areas that should be examined.

Uterine Findings

Ultrasonic evaluation of the pelvis may fail to detect the uterus. This may be explained by hysterectomy, congenital absence, elderly patient with small atrophic uterus, and inadequate urinary bladder filling. The major technical reason for inability to visualize the uterus is inadequate bladder filling, which permits air-filled small bowel loops in the pelvis to hide the uterus. It is important to evaluate the degree of bladder filling and determine if this is the reason for nonvisualization of the uterus. If the urinary bladder is only minimally distended, nonvisualization of the uterus is not a disturbing finding. If the bladder is well filled and the uterus is not seen, then close scrutiny of the bladder wall for any indentation is necessary. When no bladder indentation or uterine echoes are present, an absent uterus from whatever etiology is diagnosed. In a patient with a complete hysterectomy, the vaginal echoes end abruptly, and bowel echoes are present where the uterus should be. In a partial hysterectomy, the remaining cervical cuff may be misinterpreted as a small uterus. Congenital absence of the uterus has an appearance similar to that of a complete hysterectomy.

The prepubescent uterus has a different shape and ultrasonic appearance than the postpubescent uterus. The postpubescent uterus has a bulky fundus greater in size than the cervical region. In the prepubescent uterus, the opposite is true: the fundus is smaller in size compared to the cervical portion.

A common ultrasound request is for localization of an intrauterine device. There are several possible explanations for clinical nonvisualization of an intrauterine device: (1) the device has been expelled from the uterus, (2) it remains in the uterus and the string is not visible, (3) it has extruded into the uterine wall, or (4) it has passed through the uterine wall into the surrounding area. A combination of ultrasound and X-ray examination will resolve this problem. The ultrasonic appearance of intrauterine devices usually is quite characteristic, so that an intrauterine device is easily visualized if it is in the uterus. When it is centrally located in the body and fundus of the uterus, location within the uterine cavity is diagnosed. If the intrauterine device is eccentric in position or even partially extrauterine, then migration into the myometrium is present. If an intrauterine device is not identified on ultrasound, an x-ray examination must follow. A diagnosis of a lost intrauterine device is made if it is not present on roentgenogram; however, if the device is present roentgenographically but not found on ultrasound within the uterus, then extravasation into the surrounding area is present. It is very difficult to find an intrauterine device outside the uterus by ultrasound. The high amplitude echoes of an intrauterine device are lost in the high amplitude echoes of the surrounding bowel and adipose tissue of the pelvis.

The most common uterine masses are secondary to myomas. This entity is easily visualized with diagnostic ultrasound (Cochrane and Thomas 1974; Leopold and Asher 1975). The typical appearance is that of a rounded mass that is less echogenic than normal myometrium and much more attenuating. Occasionally, fibroids may be so lucent that they are confused for cystic masses; however, the increased attenuation of sound provides information that leads to the correct diagnosis. Fibroids may be single or multiple in number. Whenever a myoma is within the confines of the uterus, they usually do not present any diagnostic difficulties. If pedunculated and situated in the adnexal region, myomas may be misinterpreted as solid ovarian masses. This is a common dilemma in diagnostic ultrasound, and no clear cut solution is presently available.

There are certain areas of a normal uterus that may have a decreased level of echoes, suggesting the presence of fibroids. The fundus of the uterus may have lower-level echoes secondary to a thinner portion of the urinary bladder situated anteriorly. This decrease in through transmission leads to a more lucent-appearing fundus and an often mistaken diagnosis of a fundal fibroid. A second area of echo dropoff is in the cervical region, where the steep angle of the back wall of the urinary bladder decreases the transmission of sound secondary to the critical-angle phenomenon. Overdiagnosis of uterine myomas in the fundal and cervical regions is common because of these technical factors.

Myomas have a varied ultrasound appearance depending upon their anatomic structure. The common type is a relatively lucent, highly attenuating mass. When calcified, they have highly echogenic areas with acoustic shadowing posteriorly. Necrotic fibroids have irregular, central lucent regions with enhanced through transmission.

Uterine leiomyosarcomas and mixed mesodermal tumors have an ultrasonic appearance similar to degenerating fibroids. The uterus is enlarged with irregular borders, an uneven parenchymal pattern, and fluid areas from hemorrhagic necrosis. This often is accompanied by malignant ascites (Cochrane 1975; von Micsky 1977). Occasionally an ovarian malignancy invading the uterus gives a similar ultrasonic appearance. Extension of tumor into the pelvic side walls is not well visualized by ultrasound. Computed tomographic scanning is preferred for evaluating pelvic side-wall invasion.

Ovarian Masses

The ovary may have numerous masses with varied ultrasound appearances (Lawson and Albarelli 1977; Leopold and Asher 1975; Morley and Barnett 1977). Many of these masses are very characteristic in their ultrasound presentations and are readily diagnosed. This is not true of solid ovarian tumors. They usually do not have a characteristic echo pattern and can only be diagnosed as a solid ovarian lesion. Since these patients usually undergo an operation once a solid ovarian mass is diagnosed, differentiating the various solid ovarian tumors is not necessary.

A major problem facing the ultrasonographer is the diagnosis of normal ovaries; such difficulty is due to variation in size and the proximity of the distal end of the fallopian tube. If an ovary is found to be enlarged, close evaluation of ovarian parenchymal pattern will not only help detect the presence of a mass but also characterize its nature. When combined with the clinical history, such information often leads to the correct diagnosis.

The most common ovarian mass detected by ultrasound is an ovarian cyst. The ultrasound findings of an ovarian cyst are the same as for any cystic structure elsewhere in the body. Simple ovarian cysts are sonolucent masses with sharp, thin borders and enhanced through transmission. Of the various ovarian cysts, a follicular cyst is the most common. They occur during the menstrual cycle, gradually increasing in size but not exceeding 3 cm in diameter. They regress spontaneously, sometimes leaving a small amount of fluid visible in the cul-de-sac. The gradual increase in size and eventual rupture can be observed by ultrasound during the menstrual cycle. This information is helpful in determining optimal fertilization time.

A corpus luteum cyst of pregnancy is a single simple cyst commonly visualized in early pregnancy. It decreases in size with involution often occurring after 16 weeks. Theca-lutein cysts have a multiloculated appearance. They are associated with hydatidiform mole, choriocarcinoma, or multiple pregnancies. They can persist for several weeks to several months after delivery.

Theca-lutein cysts usually are fluid-filled structures with multiple septations and are greater than 3 cm in size (Fleischer, James, Krause, and Mills 1978).

Parovarian cysts are thin-walled cystic masses that can become quite large. When the urinary bladder is not distended, these large cysts are often situated low in the pelvis and confused with the urinary bladder (Haney and Trought 1978). This error of interpretation will lead to the mistaken diagnosis of a normal pelvic ultrasound in the presence of a large cystic mass.

Since normal ovaries often have numerous visible small cysts, the diagnosis of polycystic ovaries is difficult on the basis of ultrasound alone. Clinical correlation is necessary. The usual appearance of polycystic ovaries is bilaterally enlarged ovaries that are tense in appearance and oval shaped. They usually are filled with multiple thin-walled small cysts. Some of the cysts may be larger than others. These findings, in conjunction with the appropriate clinical setting, lead to the diagnosis of polycystic ovaries.

Serous and mucinous cystadenomas have a similar ultrasound appearance. They usually are thin-walled, fluid-filled cysts with several sharp curvilinear septae. Mucinous cystadenomas are septated more frequently than serous cystadenomas (Wicks, Silver, and Bree 1978). Serous and mucinous cystadenocardinomas cannot be distinguished from cystadenomas. The cystadenocarcinomas usually have a large solid component and may have malignant ascites. Cystic malignant masses of various types have thickened septae with tumor nodules projecting into the fluid-containing areas. The cyst walls are not sharply defined; the internal structure is complex; and pelvic fixation often is present (Morley and Barnett 1977; von Micsky 1977).

Solid ovarian tumors such as fibromas, fibrosarcomas, granulosa cell tumors, Brenner tumors, dysgerminomas, and malignant teratomas are not distinguishable by diagnostic ultrasound. No feature of solid tumors is characteristic except for benign teratomas, discussed later in this section. Other solid tumors have a varied ultrasound appearance more dependent on the homogeneity of the mass rather than the cell type. Ultrasound will document the presence of a solid lesion but can go no further in narrowing the diagnosis. A word of caution is in order: other entities such as chronic ectopic pregnancy, endometriosis, hemorrhage into a cyst, and pedunculated myomas will appear as solid masses on ultrasound and usually require clinical information to distinguish them from solid ovarian tumors.

Metastatic tumors of the ovary are common and originate from such primary sites as the gastrointestinal tract, other genital organs, and bronchus. These metastatic lesions may be solid or cystic in ultrasonic appearance. They are quite variable in size and may be bilateral. Since ascites often is present, the pelvis and the remainder of the abdomen should be scanned for fluid. Metastatic lesions of the ovary cannot be differentiated from other ovarian neoplasms on the basis of their ultrasound presentations (Carnovale and Samuels 1976).

Dermoids

Dermoids, or benign ovarian teratomas, are found in the young adult female and have an extremely variable appearance (Guttman 1977). They may contain fluid, fat, teeth, hair, sebaceous material, and many other structures with different ultrasonic presentations. Cystic dermoids are easily identified and appear as single or multiseptated fluid-filled cystic structures in the adnexal regions. Teeth in a dermoid appear as highly echogenic masses with acoustic shadowing and can be confused for feces in the rectosigmoid. Fat- or hair-filled dermoids are very echogenic and difficult to detect among the bowel loops in the pelvis. Because of their echogenicity, these dermoids commonly are missed on ultrasound. The only initial clue may be indentation of the urinary bladder wall. When indentation of the bladder is noted next to an echogenic and highly attenuating area, the possibility of a dermoid should be considered. Close examination often will demonstrate a small lucent rim around the echogenic area secondary to its wall. When a dermoid is suspected on ultrasound, a pelvic X-ray should be obtained. If teeth or a circular-to-oval fatty density corresponding to the size and location of the echogenic mass is identified on X-ray, a dermoid is diagnosed. When a dermoid is detected, the other ovary must be closely examined because of the likelihood of bilateral occurrence.

Pelvic Inflammatory Disease and Endometriosis

Pelvic inflammatory disease and endometriosis are two distinct and separate clinical entities with a wide range of ultrasonic appearances. Although they differ clinically, their ultrasound presentations are quite similar.

Pelvic inflammatory disease usually is bilateral except when associated with an intrauterine device. Depending on the stage of infection, there is a wide spectrum of ultrasound findings. In the acute phase, increased through transmission is present secondary to tissue edema. Sharp demarcation between the ovaries and uterus is lost secondary to inflammation. The uterus often is increased in size with a slight loss of echogenicity. These changes can return to normal over several days to weeks (Sample 1977). More severe infections, which develop into pelvic abscesses and tubo-ovarian abscesses, present as thick-walled cystic masses. In pelvic inflammatory disease as well as in endometriosis there is the general impression that these processes are filling in potential anatomic spaces rather than contained in discrete masses. In acute pelvic inflammatory disease, free fluid may be in the cul-de-sac and above the uterus.

Chronic pelvic inflammatory disease has a more solid ultrasonic appearance secondary to fibrosis and organization. This gives rise to the echogenicity present in chronic pelvic inflammatory disease. Tissue planes may be lost to the point that the uterus cannot be identified. Hydrosalpinx can result from previous infection and appears as a fluid-filled mass with sharp walls. When a dilated, fluid-filled tube is folded over on itself, the ultrasound picture is that of a multicystic mass. When any of these ultrasonic pictures are present, the possibility of pelvic inflammatory disease should be considered. Laboratory data and clinical history must then be correlated with the ultrasound findings to confirm the diagnosis of pelvic inflammatory disease.

Although endometriosis is a markedly different pathologic and clinical entity, it is quite similar to pelvic inflammatory disease in ultrasound appearance. Endometriomas may be unilateral or bilateral, single or multiple. They can range in size from a few centimeters to greater than 20 cm. Typical chocolate cysts containing lytic blood have a sonolucent appearance comparable to a simple ovarian cyst. Other endometriomas have a mixed echo appearance with fluid and solid components. Such masses are similar to abscesses or hematomas. Occasionally, they may have a solid appearance and cannot be differentiated from other solid ovarian masses (Sandler and Karo 1978). As in pelvic inflammatory disease, endometriosis tends to fill potential spaces such as the pouch of Douglas, adnexal regions, and the area cephalad to the uterus.

The ultrasound differentiation between pelvic inflammatory disease and endometriosis is difficult. When scans identify multiple sonolucent and echogenic masses with loss of tissue planes and filling in of potential anatomic spaces, pelvic inflammatory disease and endometriosis are the ultrasonographer's first considerations. Evaluation of laboratory results plus clinical history usually leads to the correct diagnosis. Other entities may have similar ultrasonic presentations and include (1) appendicitis with rupture into the pelvis, (2) chronic ectopic pregnancy, (3) posttrauma with hemorrhage into the pelvis, and (4) pelvic abscesses from various causes such as Crohn's disease or diverticulitis.

Urinary Bladder

The size, configuration, and contour of the urinary bladder were discussed in detail in the section on normal pelvic anatomy. Any distortion of bladder contour raises the possibility of an adjacent mass. The thickness of the urinary bladder wall is helpful in detecting pathology. Bladder-wall thickness often is overlooked during a pelvic ultrasound examination. When the urinary bladder is only partially filled, the wall appears evenly thickened in all borders. When markedly distended, the urinary bladder wall has a thin, sharp border except on its lateral aspects. This lack of sharpness laterally is secondary to technical factors of beamwidth and lateral resolution.

When an area of localized wall thickness is identified, the possibility of a pathologic process must be considered. Tumor, infection, and hemorrhage are the major causes of increased thickness to the urinary bladder wall. In the case of tumor, the wall often has an irregular border with an uneven echo pattern.

Masses such as stones and catheters may be seen within the bladder lumen. Urinary bladder calculi, like calculi elsewhere, are highly echogenic masses with acoustic shadowing deep to the mass. Catheters also present as intraluminal masses that vary in appearance depending on the type of catheter.

A urinary bladder diverticulum appears as a cystic mass adjacent to the urinary bladder. It usually is mistaken for a cystic mass arising from some other pelvic structure. If a bladder diverticulum is suspected, attempts are made to demonstrate its communication with the bladder. Only in this manner can the diagnosis be made by ultrasound.

References

Carnovale, R., and Samuels, B. I. Complex ovarian mass on ultrasonography: primary or metastatic tumor? (letter). *N. Engl. J. Med.* 294:446–447, 1976.

Cochrane, W. J. Ultrasound in gynecology. *Radiol. Clin. North Am.* 13:457–466, 1975.

Cochrane, W. J., and Thomas, M. A. Ultrasound diagnosis of gynecologic pelvic masses. *Radiology* 110:649–654, 1974.

Fleischer, A. C.; James, A. E., Jr.; Krause, D. A.; and Millis, J. B. Sonographic patterns in trophoblastic disease. *Radiology* 126:215–220, 1978.

Guttman, I. P., Jr. In search of the elusive benign cystic ovarian teratoma: application of the ultrasound "tip of the iceberg" sign. *J. Clin. Ultrasound* 6:403–406, 1977.

Haney, A. F., and Trought, W. S. Parovarian cysts resembling a filled urinary bladder. *J. Clin. Ultrasound* 6:53–54, 1978.

Lawson, T. L., and Albarelli, J. N. Diagnosis of gynecologic pelvic masses by gray scale ultrasonography: analysis of specificity and accuracy. *Am. J. Roentgenol.* 128:1003–1006, 1977.

Leopold, G. R., and Asher, W. M. *Fundamentals of abdominal and pelvic ultrasonography.* Philadelphia: W. B. Saunders Company, 1975, pp. 164–181.

Morley, P., and Barnett, E. The ovarian mass. In *Ultrasonography in obstetrics and gynecology,* ed. R. C. Sanders and A. E. James, Jr. New York: Appleton-Century-Crofts, 1977, pp. 333–356.

Sample, W. F. Pelvic inflammatory disease. In *Ultrasonography in obstetrics and gynecology,* ed. R. C. Sanders and A. E. James, Jr. New York: Appleton-Century-Crofts, 1977, pp. 357–385.

Sample, W. F.; Lippe, B. M.; and Gyepes, M. T. Gray-scale ultrasonography of the normal female pelvis. *Radiology* 125:477–483, 1977.

Sandler, M. A., and Karo, J. J. The spectrum of ultrasonic findings in endometriosis. *Radiology* 127:229–231, 1978.

von Micsky, L. I. Sonographic study of uterine fibromyomatoma in the non-pregnant state and during gestation. In *Ultrasonography in obstetrics and gynecology,* ed. R. C. Sanders and A. E. James, Jr. New York: Appleton-Century-Crofts, 1977, pp. 297–331.

Wicks, J. D.; Silver, T. M.; and Bree, R. L. Giant cystic abdominal masses in children and adolescents: ultrasonic differential diagnosis. *Am. J. Roentgenol.* 130:853–857, 1978.

Zemlyn, S. Comparison of pelvic ultrasonography and pneumography for ovarian size. *J. Clin. Ultrasound* 2:331–339, 1974.

CASES

Technique for Pelvic Examination

When doing a pelvic ultrasound examination, it is necessary to have the urinary bladder as distended as is comfortable for the patient. This maneuver lifts the small bowel air out of the pelvis and provides an ultrasonic window through the urine-filled urinary bladder. In women, it also elevates the pelvic organs to an area where they will be visible by the transducer beam.

The patient is examined in the supine position. Figure 178 is an example of a transverse scan obtained with the patient in the supine position. There is slight cephalad angulation of the transducer. When the urinary bladder is filled, the orientation of the uterus causes its fundus to lie somewhat anterior to the cervical area. This cephalad angulation of the transducer on transverse scans will place the sound beam more perpendicular to the long axis of the uterus. Transverse scans can be obtained with the transducer perpendicular to the patient's skin. Slight cephalad angulation, however, usually yields a better transverse examination of the uterus and adnexa.

Figure 179 is a longitudinal scan in the midline. Initially, it is useful to determine the degree of bladder filling. The transducer has a caudal angulation initially in figure 179. This gives excellent visualization of the vagina. As we reach the cervix and the uterus, the transducer continues in a more cephalad direction parallel to the long axis of the uterus.

On transverse scans, visualization of the posterior right pelvis is best obtained by scanning over the left side of the patient, as is demonstrated in figure 180. Using the bladder as an ultrasonic window, the transducer can be placed over the left side of the pelvis and angled toward the right. This will yield excellent visualization of the right pelvic wall and ovary. When examining the right ovary,

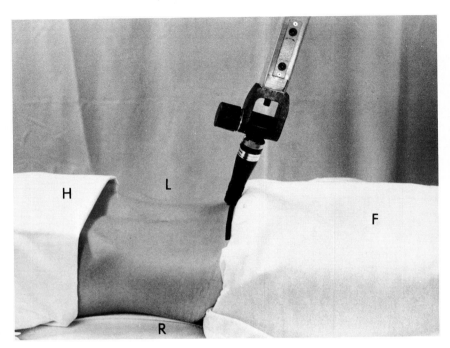

Fig. 178

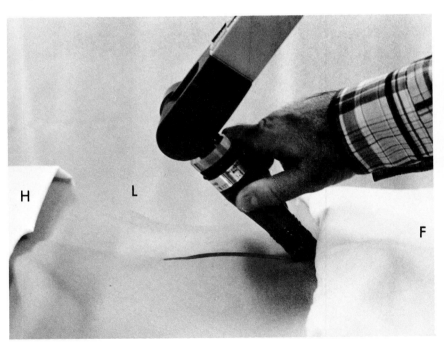

Fig. 179

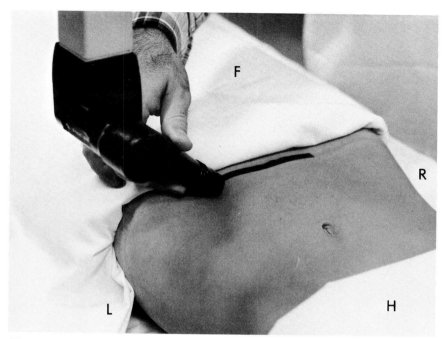

Fig. 180

a longitudinal scan should be obtained similar to that demonstrated in figure 181. Scanning the left side of the pelvis in a longitudinal plane with the transducer angled toward the right side will yield the best visualization of the right ovary in a longitudinal plane. The same is true for visualization of the left ovary. The right side of the patient is scanned with marked angulation toward the left side.

F = Foot
H = Head
L = Left
R = Right

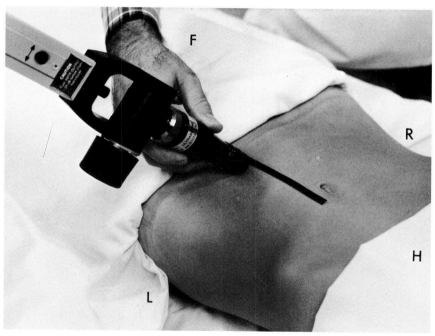

Fig. 181

Normal Longitudinal Scans   I.

When the urinary bladder is well distended, the uterus is easily visualized posterior to it. With some caudal angulation, the vagina is well seen (fig. 182). When more cephalad, the cervix and the uterus come into view. Figure 182 is an example of the normal pear-shaped appearance of the uterus with fairly even echoes throughout the myometrium. We do not see any internal echoes within the uterus on this scan. The rectum and bowel loops are noted posterior to the uterus and vagina.

Figures 183–185 are longitudinal scans of the uterus with a linear echo seen within the myometrial echoes of the uterus. This linear echo is secondary to visualization of the endometrial cavity. This is normally seen during menstruation. The linear echo is not markedly thick and has a characteristically high-amplitude echo to it. In figure 185 sonolucency is seen secondary to fluid within the vagina. This is due to urine in the vagina which is not unusual to see with marked bladder filling.

Usually, indentation in the posterior bladder wall by the fundus of the uterus can be seen. In all of these scans we see the uterine indentation on the bladder wall in the longitudinal scans.

Figure 185 also demonstrates the suggestion of a large mass posterior to the uterus. However, this is secondary to a pseudomass which is very commonly seen in pelvic studies. It is due to a duplication artifact off the urinary bladder.

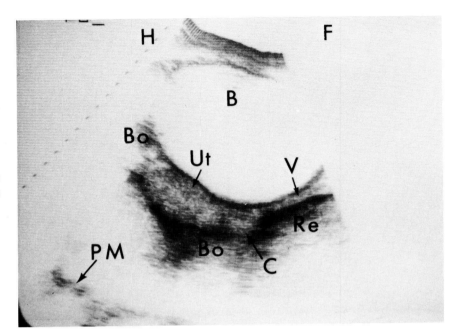

Fig. 182

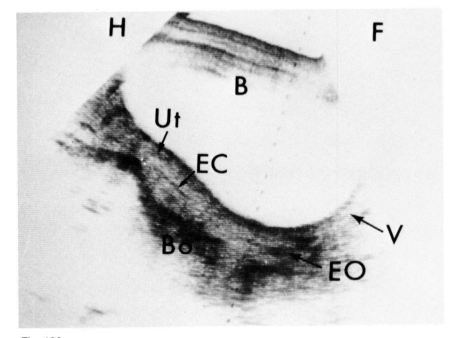

Fig. 183

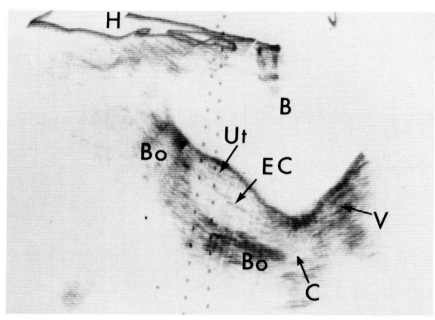

Fig. 184

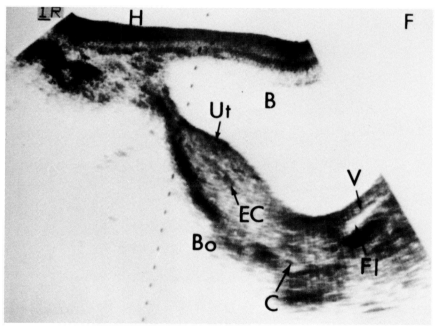

Fig. 185

B = Urinary bladder
Bo = Bowel
C = Cervix
EC = Endometrial cavity
EO = External os
F = Foot
FI = Fluid in the vagina
H = Head
PM = Pseudomass
Re = Rectum
Ut = Uterus
V = Vagina

Normal Longitudinal Scans II.

Figure 186, a longitudinal scan, demonstrates a linear echo within the uterus, secondary to visualization of the endometrial cavity. Around the endometrial cavity is a relatively sonolucent region (arrows). This usually can be visualized just prior to menstruation and may represent some edema of the uterine mucosa. A strong linear echo is also noted in the cervical region; this represents the external cervical os.

Occasionally, while scanning the uterus in the midline, an ovary in the cul-de-sac, posterior to the cervical region of the uterus, can be seen. Figure 187 is an example of an ovary in this location.

In figure 188 an ovary is seen in the midline. This time, however, it is situated superior to the fundus of the uterus. It has caused indentation (arrows) on the superior aspect of the urinary bladder. Indentation of the bladder by the uterus and ovaries is a normal occurrence. It is very important to become familiar with this indentation on the bladder wall, because it may be the only clue that a pelvic mass is present.

Figure 189 is an example of a questionable mass in the cul-de-sac region. However, it has a strong echogenic center and a relatively lucid periphery that is consistent with bowel.

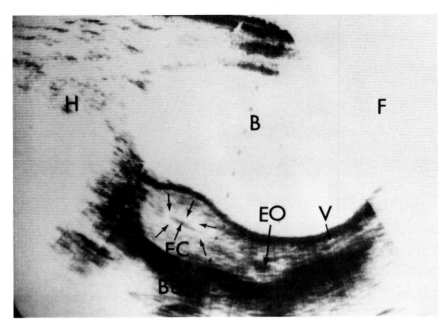

Fig. 186

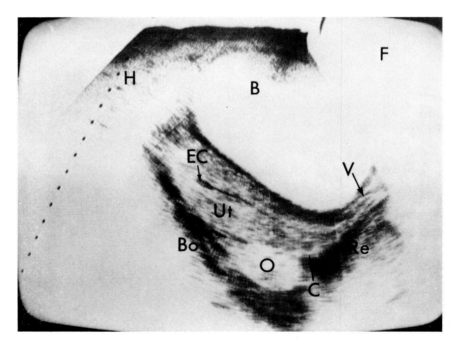

Fig. 187

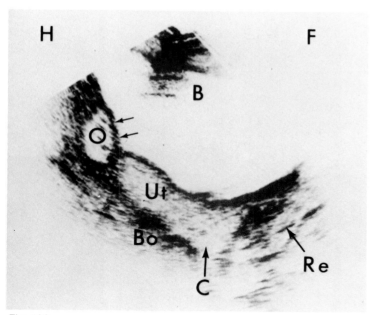

Fig. 188

Arrows = Lucencies surrounding the en-
dometrial cavity
B   = Urinary bladder
Bo   = Bowel
C   = Cervix
EC   = Endometrial cavity
EO   = External os
F   = Foot
H   = Head
O   = Ovary
Re   = Rectum
Ut   = Uterus
V   = Vagina

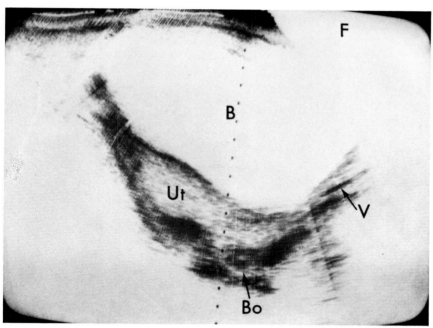

Fig. 189

Longitudinal Scans of the Normal Ovary

When examining the normal ovary, it is important to scan through the urinary bladder from the opposite side of the pelvis. For example, when scanning the right ovary, the transducer should be over the left lower abdomen and pelvis, angled toward the posterior right side of the bladder. This will yield the best visualization of the ovary on a longitudinal scan.

Figure 190 is a longitudinal scan of the right ovary. Here we see the soft echoes of the ovary situated posterior to the urinary bladder. It is important to note the indentation (arrows) of the ovary on the posterior bladder wall. This is a normal finding. As mentioned previously, indentation on the urinary bladder is important in detecting a pathological condition. Just deep to the ovary, we will see an echogenic region secondary to the piriform muscle.

In figures 191–193, several tubular structures are seen situated deep to the ovary. These tubular structures represent the internal iliac vessels. They are important landmarks and can be visualized fairly routinely. The ovary is situated anterior to them. In figure 193, we see another tubular structure situated deep to the ovary. This represents the ureter. The ovary has an oval appearance and gives a fairly homogeneous echo pattern which is often slightly less echogenic than that of the uterus.

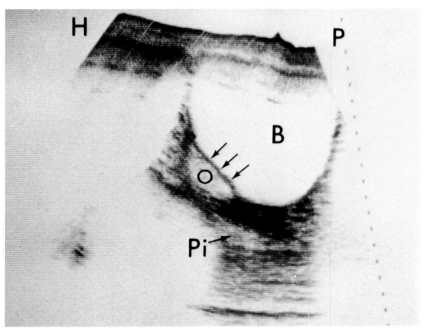

Fig. 190

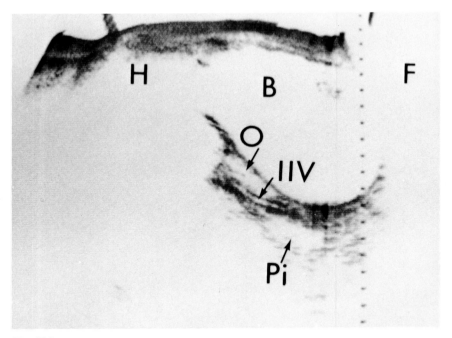

Fig. 191

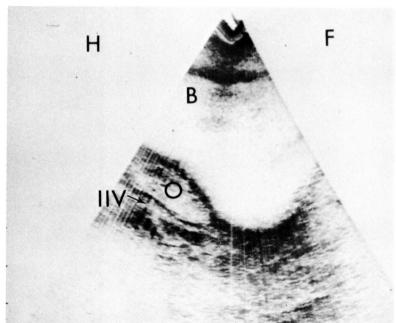

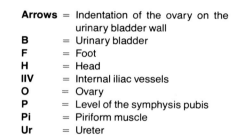

Arrows = Indentation of the ovary on the urinary bladder wall
B   = Urinary bladder
F   = Foot
H   = Head
IIV   = Internal iliac vessels
O   = Ovary
P   = Level of the symphysis pubis
Pi   = Piriform muscle
Ur   = Ureter

Fig. 192

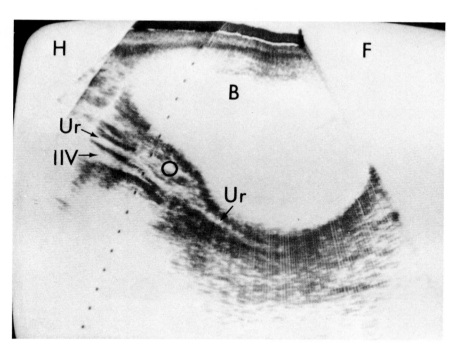

Fig. 193

Normal Transverse Scans   I.

When attempting to visualize the vagina in a transverse plane, a caudal angulation of the transducer is often necessary. Figures 194 and 195 are examples of visualization of the vagina posterior and deep to the urinary bladder. The vagina appears as a strong linear central echo surrounded by a sonolucent rim. The strong echogenic area in the vagina is due to apposition of the vaginal mucosa. Deep to the vagina are echoes often seen arising from the rectum. Scanning more cephaladly, the uterus is visualized (figs. 196 and 197). Transverse scans through the uterus are made with the transducer arm angled more cephaladly. This places the transducer beam perpendicular to the body of the uterus.

Figure 196 demonstrates linear echoes on the lateral pelvic wall, lateral to the urinary bladder. These echoes arise from the obturator internus muscle. They should not be confused with echoes arising from the ovary.

The ovary will come into view as a soft echogenic mass situated in the adnexa lateral to the uterus (fig. 197). On the left side of the uterus (fig. 197) is a highly echogenic region secondary to bowel loops, most likely the sigmoid colon. It is important to recognize the muscle planes in the pelvis so as not to confuse them with the ovary. The obturator internus muscles seen in figures 196 and 197 usually do not cause problems, because they are fairly thin and parallel the lateral urinary bladder wall.

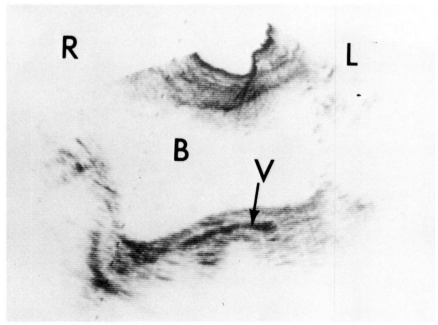

Fig. 194

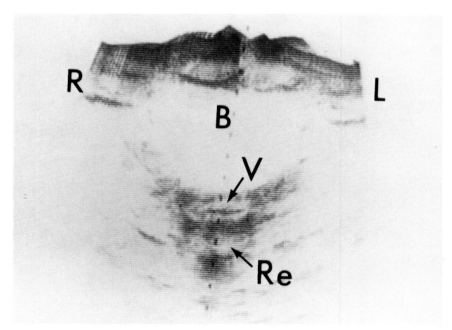

Fig. 195

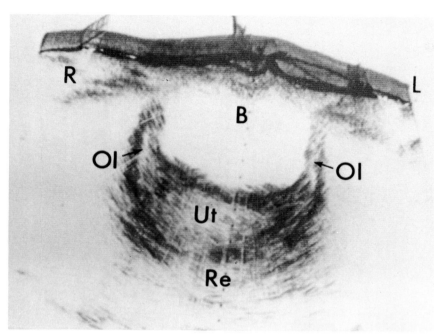

Fig. 196

B	=	Urinary bladder
Bo	=	Bowel
L	=	Left
O	=	Ovary
OI	=	Obturator internus muscle
R	=	Right
Re	=	Rectum
Ut	=	Uterus
V	=	Vagina

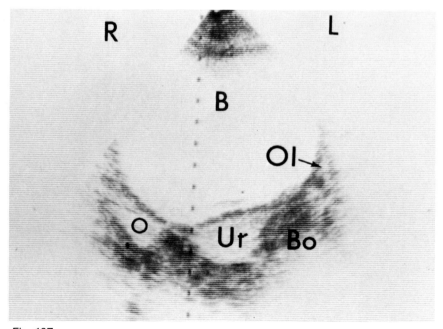

Fig. 197

Normal Transverse Scans II.

As mentioned previously, it is important to recognize the various muscle bundles within the pelvis. Figure 198 demonstrates the right obturator internus muscle lateral to the urinary bladder. Just medial to this muscle, the right ovary can be seen to the right of the uterus. The ovary is situated just medial to the obturator internus muscle in this case.

Figure 199 shows two muscle groups which occasionally may be confused with the ovary or ovarian masses. The iliopsoas muscle is seen more anterior to the left ovary in figure 199. A characteristically strong central echo is present within the iliopsoas muscle, and this makes it fairly easy to recognize. A lucent region is also noted anterior to the iliopsoas muscle; this represents the external iliac vessels. In figure 199 we visualize the piriform muscle posterior to the left ovary. It is this muscle which usually is confused for the ovary.

Figure 200 demonstrates the right piriform muscle posterior to the fallopian tube and the uterus. The piriform muscle often will be confused with the ovary. Usually symmetry between the piriform muscles can be seen, but the rectum and sigmoid will occasionally obscure the left piriform muscle, yielding only visualization of the right side. This may be confused with the ovary. If there is any question, a longitudinal scan over the region will determine whether the ovary or the muscle is visualized.

Figure 201 demonstrates a mass posterior to the uterus and secondary to an ovary which has slipped into the region of the cul-de-sac. This is a common site for the ovary. We also see the fallopian tube draping along the lateral right aspect of the uterus. Again, the characteristic appearance of the iliopsoas muscle, with the strong central echogenic center, is seen.

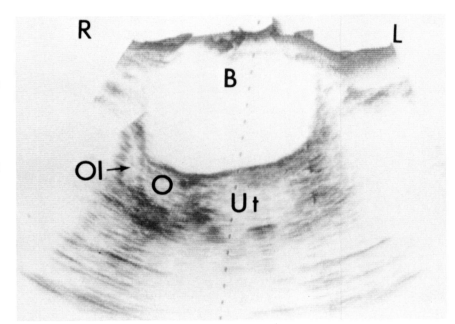

Fig. 198

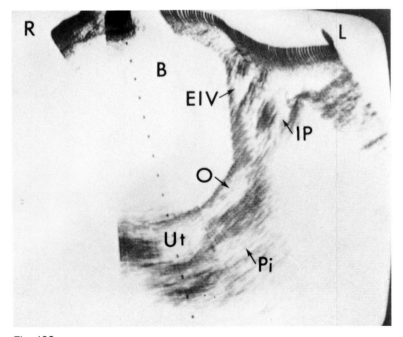

Fig. 199

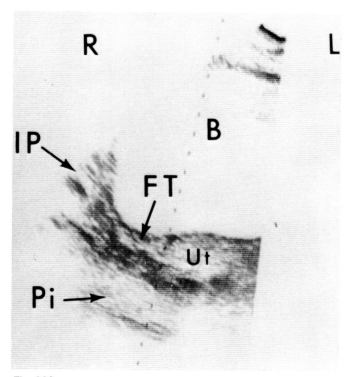

Fig. 200

B	= Urinary bladder
EIV	= External iliac vessels
FT	= Fallopian tube
IP	= Iliopsoas muscle
L	= Left
O	= Ovary
OI	= Obturator internus muscle
Pi	= Piriform muscles
R	= Right
Re	= Rectum
Ut	= Uterus

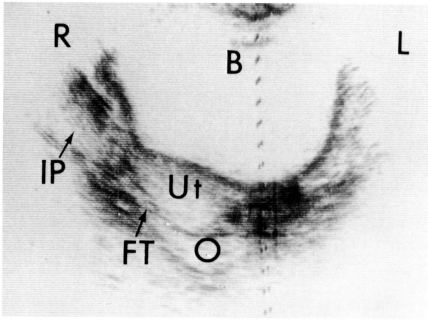

Fig. 201

Retroverted Uterus; Hysterectomy

Figure 202 is an example of a retroverted uterus. Usually the uterus is seen to parallel the superior border of the urinary bladder. However, occasionally a uterus is oriented posteriorly (fig. 202). The echoes arising from the uterus are decreased in amplitude. This is not unusual in a retroverted uterus; the sound beam is passed through the long axis of the uterus which has marked attenuation. Occasionally a myoma is misdiagnosed. It is often very difficult to diagnosis a myomatous lesion on a retroverted uterus because of this finding.

A longitudinal scan of a patient with a hysterectomy (fig. 203) is fairly characteristic of a vagina continuing posteriorly and ending abruptly without any evidence of a uterus. Superior to the vagina we see only bowel air. Occasionally, a small cervical cuff may be present and may be mistaken for a small uterus.

Figures 204 and 205 are also examples of hysterectomy, since no uterus is identified. Only bowel air is noted superior to the urinary bladder, but fluid is present in the vagina in both instances. Fluid is often seen in the vagina when doing an ultrasound examination. Most likely, it represents urine. Since the urinary bladder has to be markedly distended, the patient may be unable to avoid urinating a small amount.

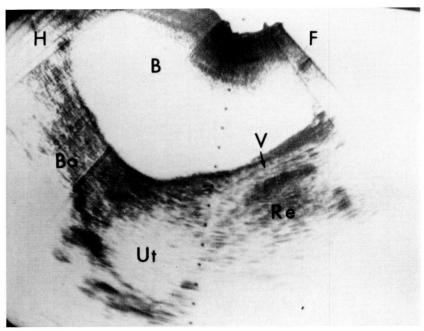

Fig. 202

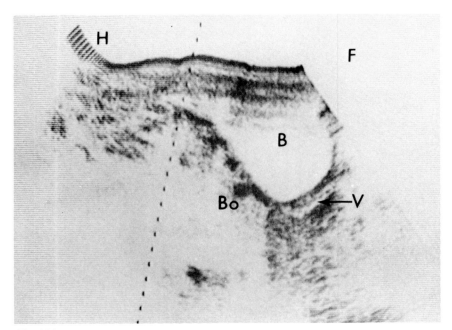

Fig. 203

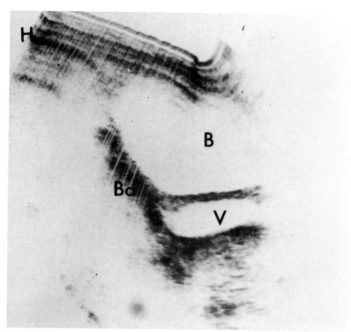

B = Urinary bladder
Bo = Bowel air
F = Foot
H = Head
Re = Rectum
Ut = Retroverted uterus
V = Vagina
v = Vagina

Fig. 204

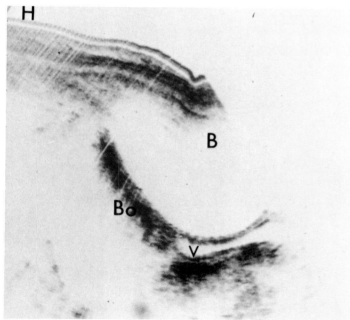

Fig. 205

Bicornuate Uterus

The patient in figures 206–209 is a 27-year-old woman who had had three pregnancies ending in a first or second trimester abortion. Because of this history, an ultrasound examination was performed, followed by a hysterosalpingogram. The diagnosis of a bicornuate uterus was made. The transverse scans (figs. 206 and 207) demonstrate myometrial echoes in the right and left pelvis consistent with a bicornuate uterus. Figure 207 is a slightly more cephalad transverse scan that shows further separation of the bicornuate uterus. The indentation on the bladder wall (arrows) by the uterus is noted. This is a normal finding in the pelvis. Posterior to the uterus are the piriform muscles which should not be mistaken for ovaries.

Figure 208 is a longitudinal scan through the long axis of the right uterus. Here we see some reverberations off the anterior wall of the urinary bladder, which is a normal finding in the pelvis. A longitudinal scan lining up the long axis of the left-sided uterus (fig. 209) demonstrates echoes within the endocervical cavity on this side. A hysterosalpingogram confirmed the diagnosis of the bicornuate uterus. This is a fairly characteristic appearance of this entity; it is best diagnosed on transverse scans through the cephalad portion of the uterus.

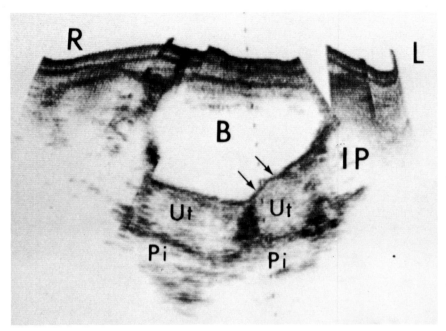

Fig. 206

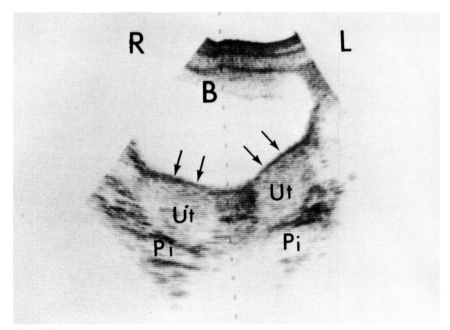

Fig. 207

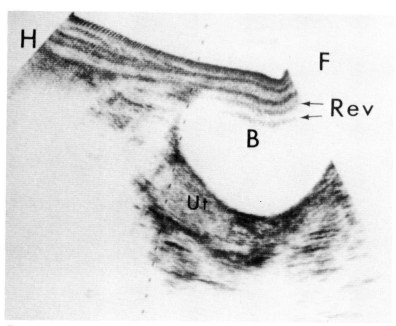

Fig. 208

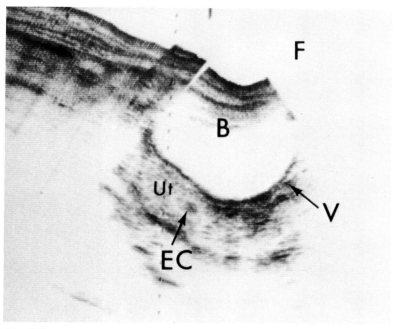

Fig. 209

Arrows	=	Indentation of the uterus on the urinary bladder wall
B	=	Urinary bladder
EC	=	Endometrial cavity
F	=	Foot
H	=	Head
IP	=	Iliopsoas muscle
L	=	Left
Pi	=	Piriform muscle
R	=	Right
Rev	=	Reverberation artifacts in the urinary bladder
Ut	=	Uterus
V	=	Vagina

Intrauterine Devices

The various intrauterine devices give fairly characteristic echo patterns within the endometrial cavity.

Figure 210 is a longitudinal scan through the uterus with a steplike appearance to the echoes arising within the endometrial cavity. This steplike appearance is characteristic of a Lippe's loop. Posterior to the central echoes is evidence of shadowing.

A longitudinal scan of the uterus (fig. 211) demonstrates a strong central echo arising from a Dalkon shield. This device presents an uninterrupted echogenic appearance without evidence of the steplike echoes noted in a Lippe's loop.

Figures 212 and 213 are longitudinal and transverse scans of a uterus containing a Copper 7 intrauterine device. Copper 7s and Copper Ts have a fairly characteristic appearance of a circular echo on transverse scans through the uterus. Longitudinal scans through the uterus show a fairly strong linear echo suggesting a small tubular structure approximately 2–3 mm in diameter.

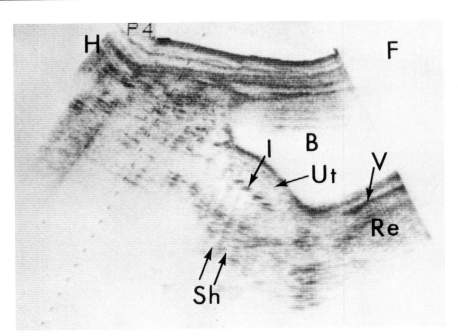

Fig. 210

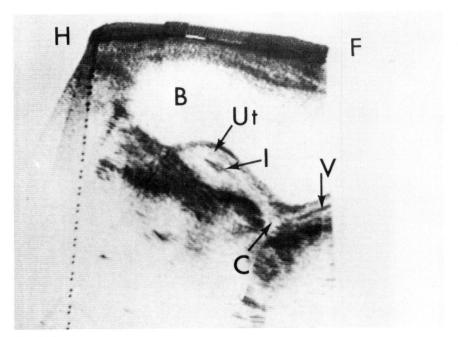

Fig. 211

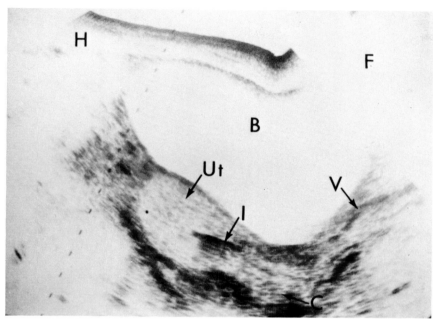

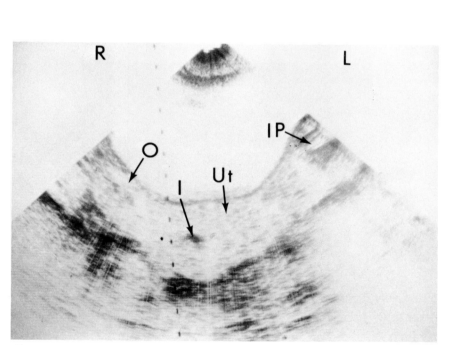

B	=	Urinary bladder
C	=	Cervix
F	=	Foot
H	=	Head
I	=	Intrauterine device
IP	=	Iliopsoas muscles
L	=	Left
O	=	Ovary
R	=	Right
Sh	=	Shadowing
Ut	=	Uterus
V	=	Vagina

Fig. 212

Fig. 213

Fibroid Uterus   I.

Leiomyomas of the uterus are fairly
common. Their appearance varies,
depending mainly upon their size. Figures 214 and 215 are of a patient
with a myoma in the posterior fundal
region of the uterus. The difference in
echogenicity between the myoma and
the normal myometrium arising from the
uterus and cervix is notable. The myoma
is less echogenic than the normal
myometrial echoes. A word of caution is
in order when evaluating the fundal region of the uterus. Very often, the fundus
of the uterus appears less echogenic
than the mid and lower uterine segments. However, this is extremely
dependent upon the degree of bladder
filling. When the urinary bladder is not
well filled, the fundal region of the uterus
often will appear less echogenic, because a distended urinary bladder is not
present anterior to it. We must remember that the through transmission from
the urinary bladder increases the level of
echoes arising from the uterus. Therefore, a misdiagnosis of a fundal myoma
is very common when the urinary
bladder is only partially filled.

Figures 216 and 217 are scans of
a myoma that contains calcification.
Calcifications are often present within a
myoma. They give very strong echoes
that are often accompanied by shadowing. The myoma in these scans yields a
less echogenic appearance as compared to the normal myometrial echoes
arising within the uterus. The transverse
scan in figure 217 shows that the
myoma is somewhat pedunculated
and situated off the posterior left
aspect of the uterus. This type is
difficult to distinguish from an
ovarian tumor.

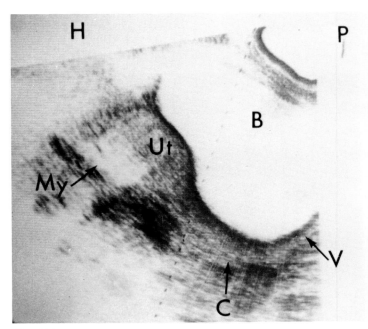

Fig. 214

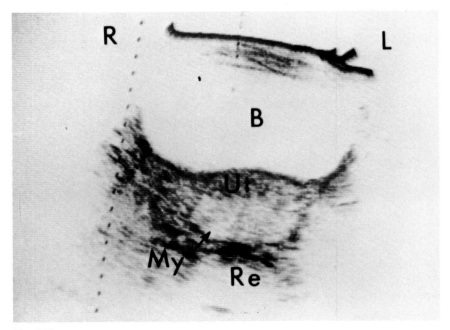

Fig. 215

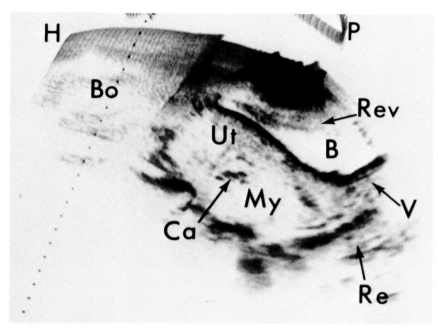

Fig. 216

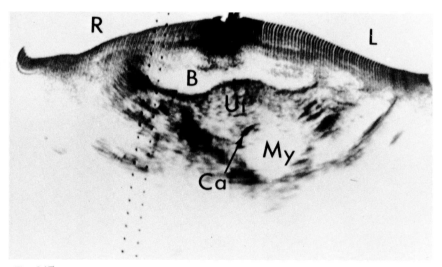

Fig. 217

B	=	Urinary bladder
Bo	=	Bowel
C	=	Cervix
Ca	=	Calcification
H	=	Head
L	=	Left
My	=	Myoma
P	=	Level of the symphysis pubis
R	=	Right
Re	=	Rectum
Rev	=	Reverberation artifacts
Ut	=	Uterus
V	=	Vagina

Fibroid Uterus   II.

Figure 218, a longitudinal scan, shows nearly the entire fundal region of the uterus containing a large myoma. The only normally appearing uterine echoes arise from the cervical region and the lower uterine segment. The myoma has a fairly homogeneous, relatively sonolucent appearance which is characteristic of a fibroid uterus.

Another longitudinal scan (fig. 219) demonstrates a uterus containing a large myoma. In this case, however, numerous echoes are present within the myoma. This is an instance of a fibroid uterus undergoing some degeneration. This can occur to such a severe degree that the uterus may occasionally be confused for a hydatidiform mole. The echoes are more irregular in a degenerating fibroid uterus than in a mole.

Figures 220 and 221 are of a patient with a large fibroid uterus, part of which was undergoing degeneration. The longitudinal scan (fig. 220) shows the myomatous uterus involving much of the entire abdomen. Again, the only normally appearing myometrial echoes are in the cervical region. There is relatively poor through transmission on the posterior aspect of the myoma, and this is another characteristic of fibroid lesions within the uterus. Figure 221 is a transverse scan of a myomatous mass with attenuation on the right side. The portion of the mass on the left side, however, does have some through transmission with a relatively sonolucent central area. This is due to fluid present within a degenerating fibroid uterus. When severe degeneration occurs, a myoma may appear relatively echo-free with through transmission secondary to fluid within its central portion.

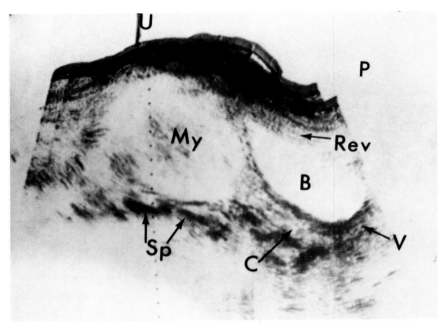

Fig. 218

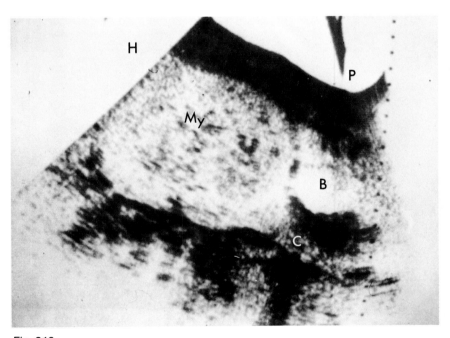

Fig. 219

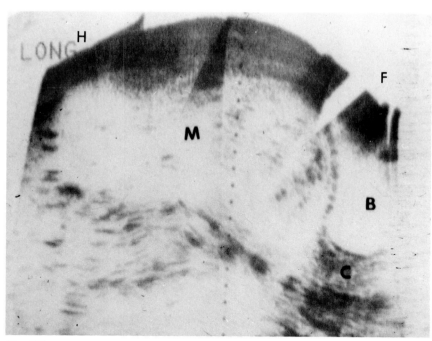

Fig. 220

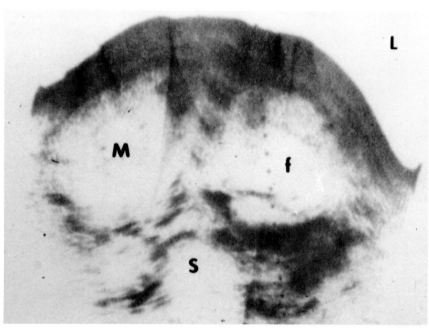

Fig. 221

Cervical Carcinoma; Mixed Mesodermal Sarcoma of the Uterus

Figures 222–224 are ultrasound scans of a patient with cervical carcinoma. Figure 222 is a longitudinal scan with a less echogenic cervical region which is also the site of the cervical carcinoma. The difference in echogenicity between the uterus and the cervix can be noted. The cervix is markedly enlarged with somewhat irregular borders, along with decreased echo amplitude. Figure 223 is a transverse section through the cervix in which we again see decreased echogenicity to the cervical carcinoma. Figure 224 is a transverse section, higher and through the normal portion of the uterus. We can note the normally appearing echo pattern of the myometrium in the uninvolved portion of the uterus. The decreased echogenicity in the cervical region is not specific for cervical carcinoma and could represent a cervical fibroid.

Figure 225 is a longitudinal scan of the pelvis and lower abdomen of a 58-year-old woman. Here we see enlargement of the uterus. The echogenicity of the uterus is somewhat irregular. Although this could represent involvement of the uterus with fibroids, a carcinoma of the uterus or other malignancy could not be ruled out. At surgery, a mixed mesodermal sarcoma of the uterus with numerous tumor implants throughout the pelvis was found.

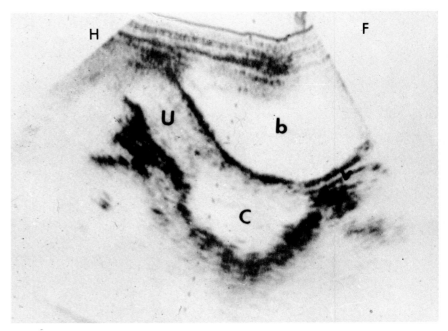

Fig. 222

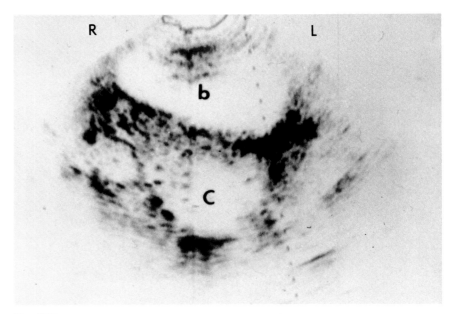

Fig. 223

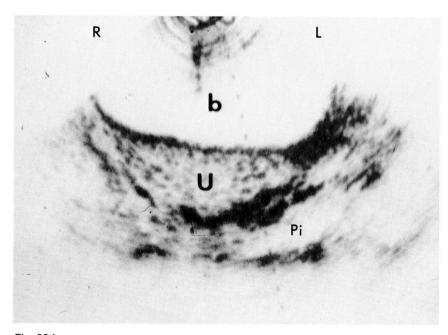

Fig. 224

SOURCE: The case in figure 225 is provided through the courtesy of Dr. B. Green, M. D. Anderson Hospital, Texas Medical Center, Houston, Texas.

b	=	Urinary bladder
C	=	Cervical carcinoma
F	=	Foot
H	=	Head
L	=	Left
Pi	=	Piriform muscle
R	=	Right
U	=	Uterus
Ut	=	Mixed mesodermal sarcoma of the uterus
V	=	Vagina

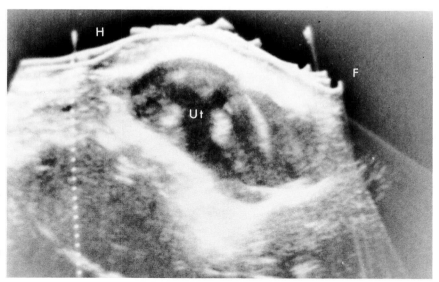

Fig. 225

Uterine Neoplasms

Figures 226 and 227 are scans of a 66-year-old woman with lower-abdominal pain and a palpable pelvic mass. Ultrasound examination demonstrated a large mass within the pelvis and lower abdomen. The echogenic portion of this mass was noted posterior to a sonolucent segment and was felt to be fluid. At surgery, adenocarcinoma of the endometrium was diagnosed. The ultrasound examination demonstrated evidence of necrosis of the tumor with fluid anteriorly and through transmission and echogenicity posteriorly. Uterine carcinoma is difficult to distinguish from a necrotic fibroid, but uterine carcinomas appear to undergo necrosis somewhat more frequently than fibroids.

Figures 228 and 229 are of an elderly woman admitted for severe pelvic pain and fever. The patient had a previous diagnosis of a large uterine mixed mesodermal sarcoma. The pelvic pain developed following radiation therapy. Ultrasound examination demonstrated an enlarged uterus. In the central and anterior portion of the uterus, a relatively sonolucent mass indicates the presence of fluid. At surgery, this turned out to be a necrotic abscess within a uterine mesodermal sarcoma. Again, uterine enlargement with fluid is present, indicating necrosis, hemorrhage, or abscess.

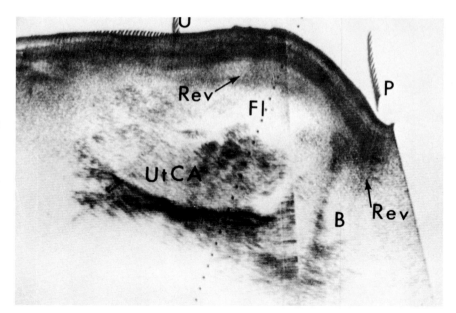

Fig. 226

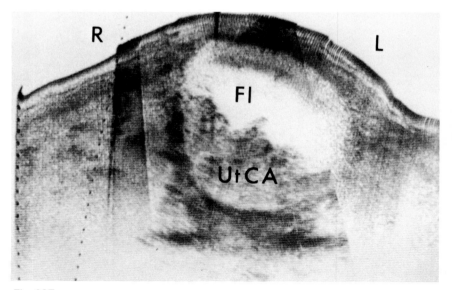

Fig. 227

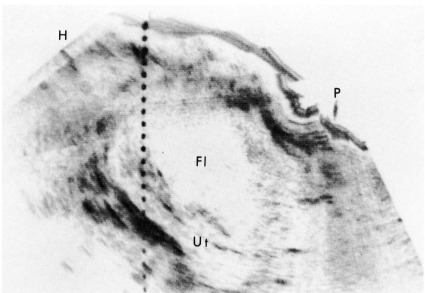

Fig. 228

SOURCE: The case for figures 228 and 229 is provided through the courtesy of Dr. B. Green, M. D. Anderson Hospital, University of Texas Medical Center, Houston, Texas.

B	= Urinary bladder
Fl	= Necrotic fluid
H	= Head
L	= Left
P	= Level of the symphysis pubis
R	= Right
Rev	= Reverberations
U	= Umbilical level
Ut	= Uterus
UtCA	= Adenocarcinoma of the uterus

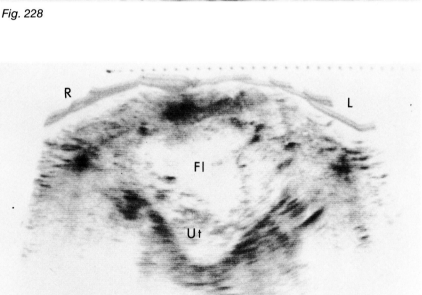

Fig. 229

Ovarian Cysts

Functional follicular cysts are encountered quite often during an ultrasound examination of the female pelvis. They can range in size from a few millimeters to large masses. The simple cysts have sonolucent centers with good through transmission and sharp borders. They usually do not cause any diagnostic problems or become confused with such things as abscesses, hematomas, or necrotic tumors. We look for the sharp borders and good through transmission to confirm the diagnosis of a simple ovarian cyst. A simple ovarian cyst seen on one examination will often disappear. We often see fluid in the cul-de-sac following spontaneous rupture of an ovarian cyst. This is a common finding.

Figure 230 is a transverse scan of a patient with a small 2-cm cyst of the right ovary. The left ovary is in the normal position. Just posterior to the left ovary and lateral to the uterus is a strong circular echogenic region which represents bowel. This often may be confused with an ovarian mass, especially with a dermoid. The echoes behind the ovarian cyst are of very high amplitude when compared to the echoes behind the left ovary. This is consistent with its fluid-filled nature.

A longitudinal scan of a different patient (fig. 231) demonstrates an ovarian cyst in the central portion of the ovary. Here we see the ovarian cyst is only 1 cm in size, but it stands out quite easily as a sonolucent mass within the soft echoes of the normal ovarian parenchyma. The strong border surrounding the ovarian cyst is fairly characteristic of a simple cyst.

Figures 232 and 233 are from a patient with a functional ovarian cyst of the left ovary. A transverse scan (fig. 232) demonstrates a sonolucent mass in the left adnexa, consistent with an ovarian cyst. Very strong echoes are seen posterior to the ovarian cyst, indicating through transmission. This may, however, be difficult to evaluate in many instances because of the strong echoes which arise from air-filled bowel. Numerous curvilinear strong echoes secondary to reverberations off a strong air-filled bowel interface are present on the left

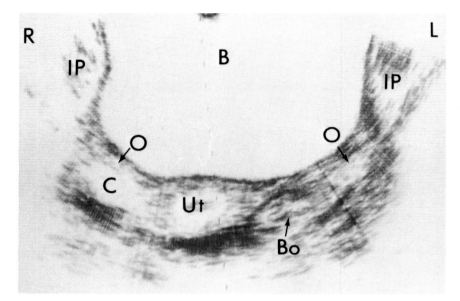

Fig. 230

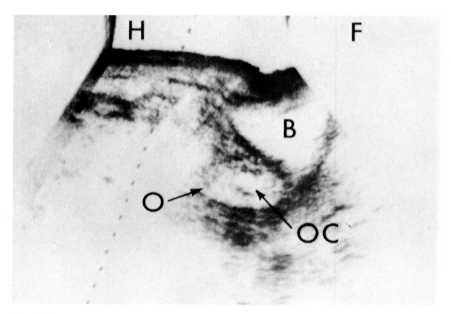

Fig. 231

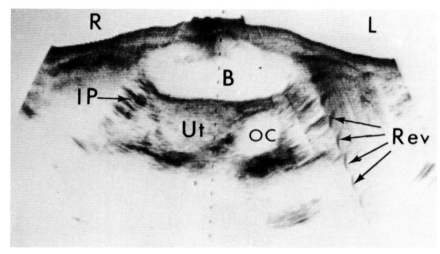

Fig. 232

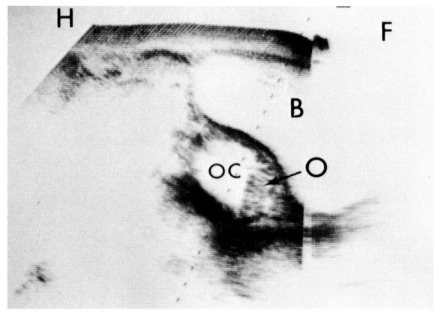

Fig. 233

side of the abdomen. This is a fairly common artifact in the pelvis. Figure 233 is a longitudinal scan of the same patient with the superior half of the ovary completely fluid-filled by the ovarian cyst. The caudal half of the ovary has a normal echogenic pattern to it consistent with a normal ovarian parenchyma. The indentation of the left ovary on the posterior aspect of the bladder wall is notable. This indentation becomes extremely important in evaluating pelvic masses, as will be shown in the following cases.

B	=	Urinary bladder
Bo	=	Bowel
C	=	Ovarian cyst
F	=	Foot
H	=	Head
IP	=	Iliopsoas muscles
L	=	Left
O	=	Ovaries
OC	=	Ovarian cyst
R	=	Right
Rev	=	Reverberation artifacts
Ut	=	Uterus

Ovarian Cysts—
Hemorrhagic and
Theca-Lutein

Figure 234 is a longitudinal scan of a left ovary with a small 1-cm cyst in its superior portion. This is an excellent example of visualization of the ovary anterior to the internal iliac vessels. We often have difficulty locating the ovary on longitudinal scans unless the internal iliac vessels can be visualized. The normal parenchymogram of the ovary can be seen in the caudal portion with the sonolucent ovarian cyst present in the cephalad portion.

Figure 235 is a transverse scan of a patient with a large right adnexal mass which was not completely sono-lucent. It eventually was found to be a hemorrhagic ovarian cyst. The large right adnexal mass is sonolucent ante-riorly and represents a fluid-filled ovarian cyst. We see soft echoes on the posterior aspect of the mass as well as a fluid–fluid level secondary to hemor-rhage. An indentation on the posterior right bladder floor (arrows) is a con-sistent finding in large pelvic masses. Studying the bladder floor superior to the uterus a similar, although less dra-matic, indentation is seen. Whenever pelvic masses are easy to identify, the bladder floor finding is not critical. When echogenic masses blend into the strong echoes of the bowel-filled pelvis, how-ever, the indentation on the bladder floor can become extremely important.

Figures 236 and 237 are of a 24-year-old woman whose uterus had been evacuated for a hydatidiform mole 1 week prior to the ultrasound examina-tion. After evacuation of the uterus, she was still found to have a pelvic and abdominal mass. Scans performed at that time demonstrated multiple fluid-filled sonolucent masses in the pelvis and lower abdomen (figs. 236 and 237). A multiloculated appearance to the mass is demonstrated here, with numerous curvilinear echoes separat-ing the sonolucent fluid-filled areas. In figure 237, the uterus is seen posterior to the urinary bladder and separate from these fluid-filled masses. Theca-lutein cysts which are associated with hyda-tidiform moles were diagnosed. The

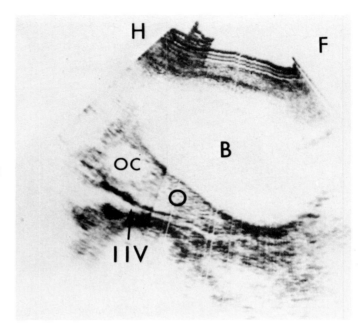

Fig. 234

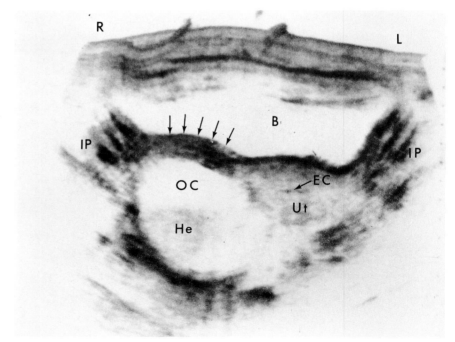

Fig. 235

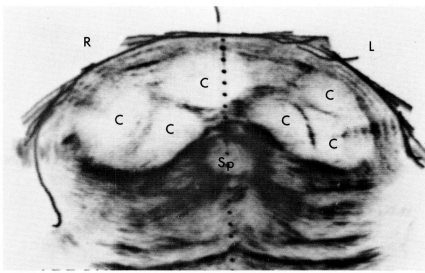

Fig. 236

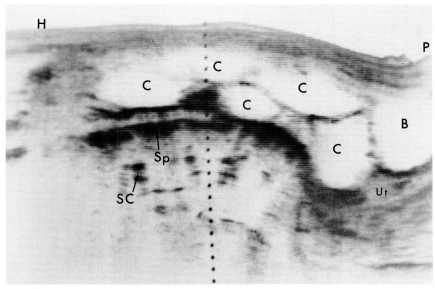

Fig. 237

multiloculated appearance cannot be distinguished from numerous such other entities as cystadenomas.

SOURCE: The case for figure 235 is provided through the courtesy of Dr. R. Bree, Toledo Hospital, Toledo, Ohio. The case for figures 236 and 237 is provided through the courtesy of Dr. B. Green, M. D. Anderson Hospital, Texas Medical Center, Houston, Texas.

B	=	Urinary bladder
C	=	Theca-lutein cyst
EC	=	Endometrial cavity
F	=	Foot
H	=	Head
He	=	Hemorrhage in an ovarian cyst
IIV	=	Internal iliac vessels
IP	=	Iliopsoas muscles
L	=	Left
O	=	Ovary
OC	=	Ovarian cyst
P	=	Level of the symphysis pubis
R	=	Right
SC	=	Spinal canal
Sp	=	Spine
Ut	=	Uterus

Polycystic Ovaries

Figures 238–241 are pelvic ultrasound scans of a 16-year-old girl referred for secondary amenorrhea. Examination was concentrated on the ovaries to determine their size and echogenicity. A longitudinal scan in the midline (fig. 238) shows the uterus to be of normal size and stimulated. A stimulated uterus has a fundal region that is usually thicker and larger than the cervical region. The unstimulated uterus will have a small thin fundus with a smaller diameter than the cervical region.

A large sonolucent mass is also present posterior to the urinary bladder. This is a false mass (arrows) and secondary to an artifact. The duplication artifact of the urinary bladder can present as a false mass. This is a fairly common occurrence, and care must be taken not to misdiagnosis an extremely large sonolucent mass in the pelvis. The patient must return with varying bladder filling if any question of a false mass has been created by bladder duplication. In trying to find the ovaries, we can often follow the uterus until the fallopian tubes are visualized. A transverse scan (fig. 239) demonstrates the fallopian tubes quite well bilaterally. The piriform muscles could be confused for the ovaries on this patient. They are, however, situated somewhat posterior to the uterus and are fairly symmetrical in appearance. We see only the anterior and posterior borders of the piriform muscles, not the lateral borders.

Following the fallopian tubes, the ovaries can finally be identified bilaterally. A transverse scan (fig. 240), that is actually cephalad to the fundus of the uterus shows the uterus to be no longer in the central portion of the scan. Bowel gas is seen. If the fallopian tubes had not been followed, the piriform muscles in figure 239 might have been misinterpreted as the ovaries. In figure 240 we see the ovaries bilaterally. The right ovary is anterior to the internal iliac vessels. On this transverse scan, the ovaries have a much coarser appearance than those noted in previous examples. Numerous strong linear echoes are present within them.

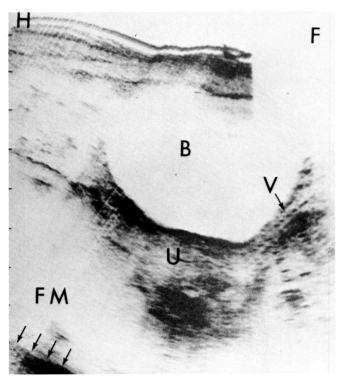

Fig. 238

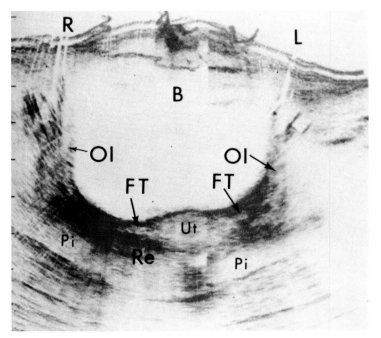

Fig. 239

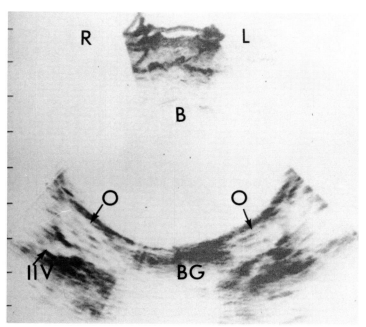

Fig. 240

Figure 241 is a longitudinal scan of the right ovary, which is seen anterior to the internal iliac vessels. Again, numerous curvilinear strong echoes within the ovary are noted. These are consistent with the walls of the numerous small cysts in these polycystic ovaries. The cysts are quite small in size. The lumen cannot actually be visualized but the sharp echogenic walls are demonstrated. This is fairly characteristic of polycystic ovaries. The patient also had hormonal levels which confirmed the diagnosis of polycystic disease.

B	=	Urinary bladder
BG	=	Bowel gas
F	=	Foot
FM and arrows	=	False mass due to bladder duplication artifact
FT	=	Fallopian tubes
H	=	Head
IIV	=	Internal iliac vessels
L	=	Left
O	=	Ovaries
OI	=	Obturator internus muscles
Pi	=	Piriform muscles
R	=	Right
Re	=	Rectum
U	=	Uterus
Ut	=	Uterus
V	=	Vagina

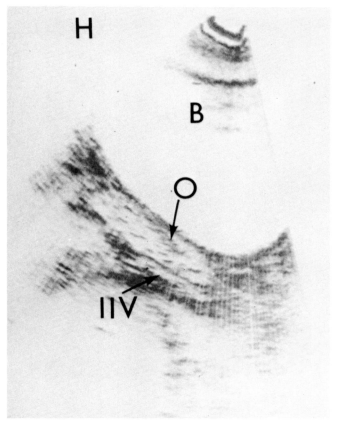

Fig. 241

Mucinous Cystadenocarcinoma; Papillary Serous Cystadenocarcinoma

Figures 242 and 243 are scans of a 62-year-old woman with increasing abdominal distention. An intravenous pyelogram demonstrated no obstruction of the ureters; however, there was a soft-tissue density over the abdomen. Ultrasound examination demonstrated a multiloculated mass (figs. 242 and 243). It is a large mass with numerous fluid-filled areas separated by curvilinear echoes. This finding is fairly characteristic of a cystadenoma or cystadenocarcinoma of the ovaries. At surgery, a large 20-cm mass was found. Also present were numerous metastatic implants throughout the abdomen with nodules over the diaphragm, liver, gallbladder, right kidney, stomach, and omentum. The pathology report on this mass was mucinous cystadenocarcinoma. Mucinous and serous cystadenocarcinomas have a fairly similar appearance and cannot be distinguished with ultrasound. They present as a multiloculated fluid-filled mass with numerous curvilinear echoes within it.

Figures 244 and 245 are from another patient with an ultrasound examination demonstrating both a solid (arrows) and a fluid component to a rather large pelvic mass. This mixed-echo pattern is more suspicious for carcinoma because of the large solid component present within the mass. At surgery, it was found to be a papillary serous cystadenocarcinoma.

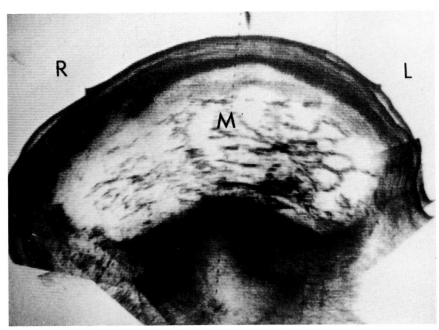

Fig. 242

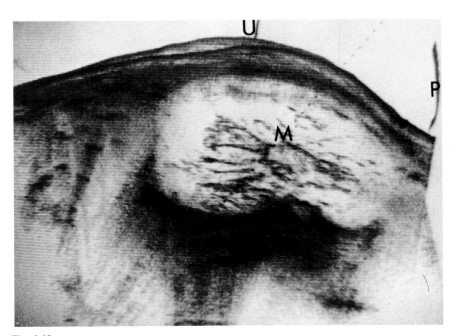

Fig. 243

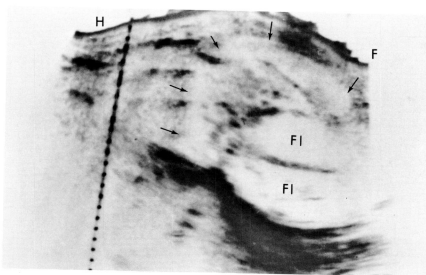

Fig. 244

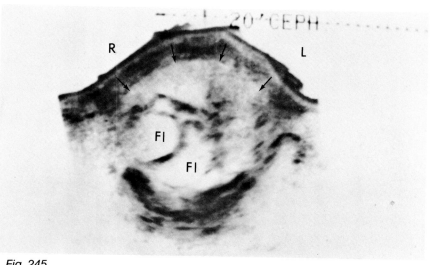

Fig. 245

SOURCE: The case for figures 242 and 243 was provided through the courtesy of Dr. B. Green, M. D. Anderson Hospital, University of Texas Medical Center, Houston, Texas.

Arrows	=	Solid component to a papillary serous cystadenocarcinoma
F	=	Foot
Fl	=	Fluid component to the mass
H	=	Head
L	=	Left
M	=	Mucinous cystadenocarcinoma
P	=	Level of the symphysis pubis
R	=	Right
U	=	Umbilical level

Papillary Cystadenocarcinoma

Figures 246–249 are scans of a 14-year-old girl with increasing abdominal girth. An intravenous pyelogram was initially performed, and it indicated a suggestion of small bowel obstruction with areas of decreased density noted over the abdomen. Because of this, an ultrasound examination was done. This case is quite interesting in that it shows the various presentations of a cystadenocarcinoma. Figure 246 is a longitudinal scan of the abdomen and pelvis from the xyphoid to the symphysis pubis. Ascitic fluid is seen beneath the liver and in the pelvis. In figure 249 ascitic fluid is seen in the pelvis surrounding the uterus. Also noted in figures 246 and 249 is a large echogenic mass just above the ascitic fluid in the pelvis. It has a fairly homogeneous echogenic component to it, indicating the solid nature of this tumor.

A second component in this mass, however, is a more characteristic appearance of a cystadenocarcinoma. This is in the mid and upper abdomen. In figures 246, 247, and 248, numerous curvilinear echoes surrounding fluid-filled regions are noted. A transverse scan (fig. 248) of the midabdomen demonstrates the solid component of the mass along with the fluid and curvilinear echoes. In fact, the fluid-filled areas are highly suggestive of bowel loops, with which this entity could be confused. In papillary cystadenocarcinoma, however, the fluid-filled masses appear somewhat more irregular and disorganized than bowel loops. Also noted in figures 247 and 248, is ascitic fluid in the right lateral gutter of the abdomen. At surgery, this mass was found to be a papillary cystadenocarcinoma. It had a large solid component in its inferior portion and a more characteristic fluid-filled component in the cephalad region.

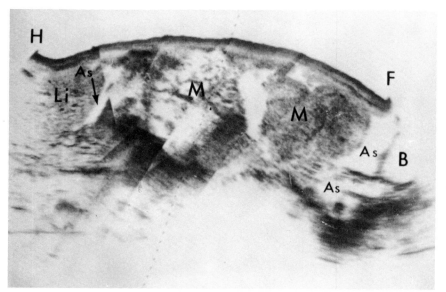

Fig. 246

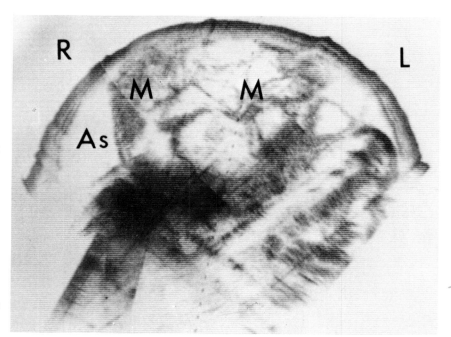

Fig. 247

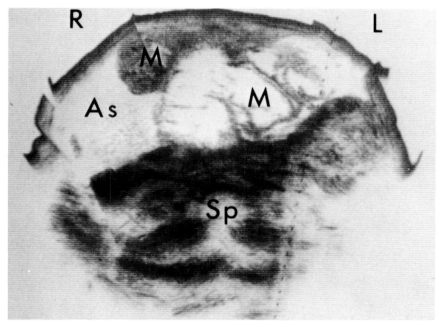

As = Ascites
B = Urinary bladder
F = Foot
H = Head
L = Left
Li = Liver
M = Papillary cystadenocarcinoma
R = Right
Sp = Spine
Ut = Uterus

Fig. 248

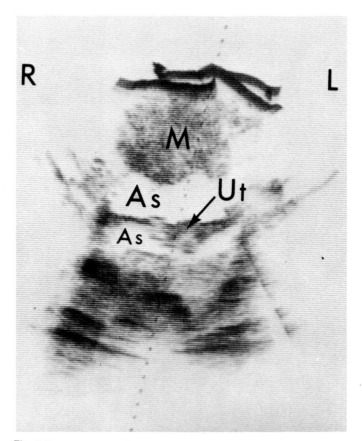

Fig. 249

Solid Ovarian Tumors

Solid ovarian tumors give an ultrasonic appearance of large echogenic masses within the pelvis. The ultrasonic appearance, however, is not very helpful in distinguishing one type of tumor from another. The major difficulty with a pelvic ultrasound examination of a solid ovarian tumor is the inability to distinguish it as separate from the uterus. If a complete separation of the uterus from the solid mass can be shown, an adnexal lesion can be diagnosed. If the lesion cannot be separated entirely from the uterus, however, the possibility of a uterine growth must be considered.

Figure 250 is a longitudinal scan that demonstrates a large mass superior to the uterus. The mass is markedly attenuating (arrows). The posterior wall of the mass is difficult to see because of this marked attenuation. The possibility of a pedunculated fibroid off the fundus of the uterus cannot definitely be ruled out. A fairly good interface is seen between the mass and the uterus. This mass turned out to be a fibrosarcoma of the ovary. Fibrous tumors of the ovary can yield an ultrasonic appearance similar to that of fibroids of the uterus. The architecture of the tumor is usually fairly sonolucent with marked attenuation and poor through transmission, as is seen in a fibroid of the uterus.

Figure 251 is a longitudinal scan of a 10-year-old girl with a pelvic mass. Here we see a large sonolucent mass, separate from the uterus. Although the mass is extremely sonolucent, there is very poor through transmission deep to it. This may be confused for a cystic lesion. The lack of an extremely sharp posterior border and through transmission, however, indicates its solid nature by ultrasound. At exploration, a 10 x 5 x 3 cm, solid lobulated mass of the left ovary was found. It was diagnosed as a fibrosarcoma of the left ovary. Again, fibrous lesions of the ovary can be fairly sonolucent masses with poor through transmission similar to fibroid lesions of the uterus.

Figure 252 is a longitudinal scan of the pelvis of an 8-year-old girl with acute lymphocytic leukemia. A large, relatively lucent mass is seen posterior to the

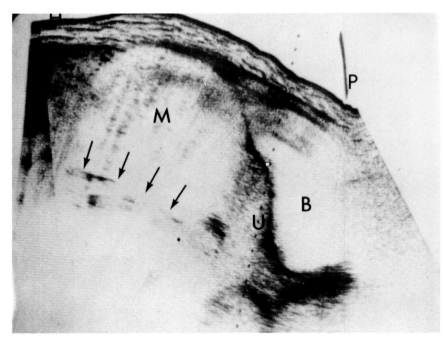

Fig. 250

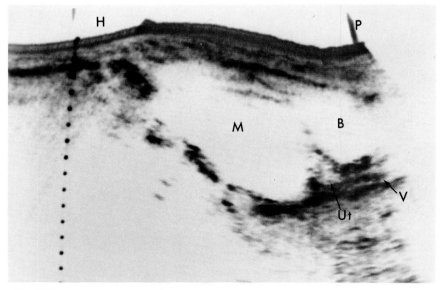

Fig. 251

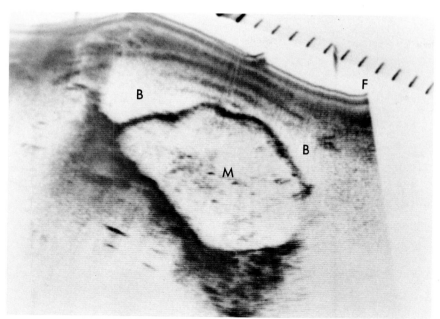

Fig. 252

urinary bladder. A marked irregular indentation on the posterior wall of the urinary bladder is also noted. Diffuse echoes are present within the mass, indicating the solid nature of this lesion. It turned out to be leukemic ovarian infiltrates.

Figure 253 is a longitudinal scan of the pelvis of a 27-year-old woman with increasing abdominal girth. Ultrasound demonstrated a large echogenic mass of the pelvis and abdomen. The distention of the abdominal wall by this mass can be seen. The solid nature was confirmed by numerous internal echoes and a poorly defined posterior wall with a lack of through transmission. This was found to be a dysgerminoma of the ovary. These rapidly growing tumors of the ovary cannot be distinguished by their ultrasonic appearance.

SOURCE: Figures 251 and 252 are provided through the courtesy of Dr. B. Green, M. D. Anderson Hospital, Texas Medical Center, Houston, Texas.

A	=	Aorta
Arrows	=	Lack of through transmission
B	=	Urinary bladder
F	=	Foot
H	=	Head
M	=	Solid ovarian mass
P	=	Level of the symphysis pubis
U	=	Uterus
Ut	=	Uterus
V	=	Vagina

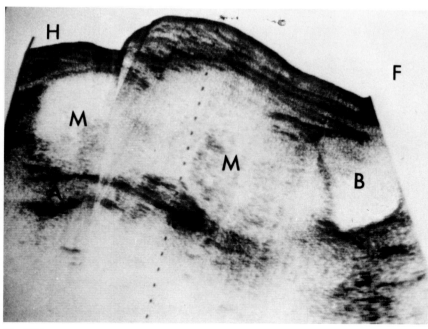

Fig. 253

Dysgerminoma

Figures 254 and 255 are ultrasound examinations of a 15-year-old girl with increased abdominal girth. Ultrasound examination demonstrated a large solid mass in the pelvis and abdomen. The anterior abdominal wall is distended secondary to the size of the mass. Within the mass are numerous strong echoes (arrows) which are of very high amplitude. An abdominal film demonstrated scattered calcifications throughout the abdomen, corresponding to these highly echogenic regions within the mass. Surgery demonstrated that this was a dysgerminoma. These tumors can grow extremely rapidly. They give an ultrasonic appearance of a solid lesion within the pelvis and abdomen.

Figures 256 and 257 are scans of a patient with dysgerminoma. This 13-year-old girl had had a large 20-cm dysgerminoma removed from the right ovary 1 year previously. Figure 256 is a transverse scan of the patient several months after surgery. The uterus is seen deviated slightly to the right. A mass in the left adnexal region represents the left ovary. The posterior left wall of the urinary bladder is seen to have a normal contour. The echogenicity of the ovary was somewhat worrisome at that time. It was decided to follow the patient serially with ultrasound examinations.

Figure 257 is a transverse scan of the same patient approximately 4 months after the exam in figure 256. We now see an enlargement of the left adnexal mass. An indentation present on the left posterior urinary blader wall (arrows) is also noted. Evaluation of the bladder wall is an excellent means for detecting pelvic masses or changes in any pelvic masses. Although this depends on the degree of bladder filling, it can provide important diagnostic information. The left ovary is now enlarged (fig. 257). An irregular echo pattern throughout it indicates a solid lesion. The patient was also found to have a dysgerminoma of the left ovary.

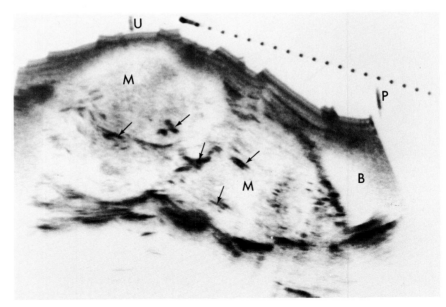

Fig. 254

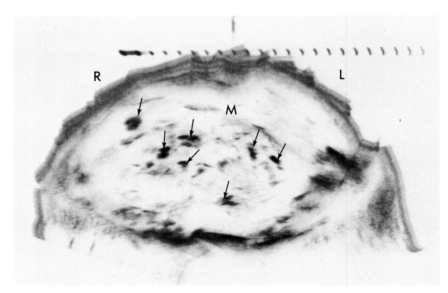

Fig. 255

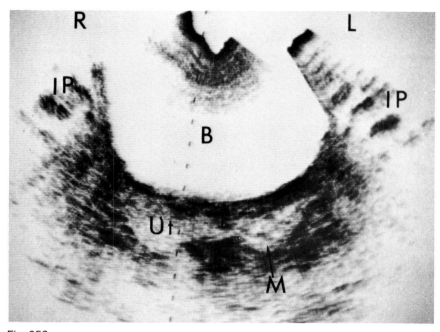

Fig. 256

SOURCE: The case for figures 254 and 255 is provided through the courtesy of Dr. B. Green, M. D. Anderson Hospital, Texas Medical Center, Houston, Texas.

Arrows	=	Areas of calcification in the dysgerminoma (figs. 254 and 255)
Arrows	=	Indentation on the bladder wall (fig. 257)
B	=	Urinary bladder
IP	=	Iliopsoas muscle
L	=	Left
M	=	Dysgerminoma
P	=	Level of the symphysis pubis
R	=	Right
U	=	Umbilical level
Ut	=	Uterus

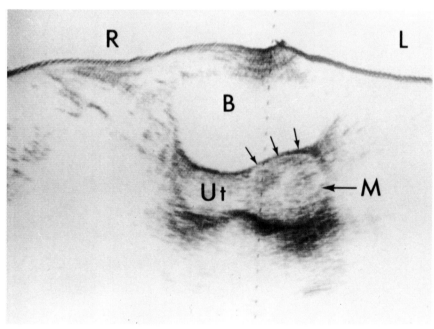

Fig. 257

Dermoids I.

Teratomas of the ovary can give various ultrasonic appearances. They can be entirely cystic, highly echogenic, or a mixture of the two.

Figure 258 is a longitudinal scan of a 14-year-old girl who underwent exploratory surgery for removal of a large pelvic mass. The ultrasonic findings were a large fluid-filled mass secondary to a cystic dermoid. This extended from the top of the urinary bladder to the xyphoid level. The cystic dermoid was found to contain 8000 cc of yellowish fluid. Cystic dermoids, which are mainly fluid-filled, present as a sonolucent mass within the pelvis or abdomen, similar to other ovarian cysts. This is an example of a dermoid filling the entire abdomen.

Figures 259–261 are ultrasound scans of a 48-year-old woman who noticed a slight increase in abdominal girth five years earlier. There was progressive increase in abdominal size through the years, with a sudden rapid increase approximately 1 year before. Four months prior to admission, she noticed the onset of pain and a further increase in size of the abdomen. When she finally entered the hospital, an ultrasound examination revealed an extremely confusing picture. A longitudinal scan (fig. 259) demonstrates a solid component to the mass adherent to the anterior abdominal wall. The abdomen is filled with fluid with the uterus and bowel loops floating within it. Figure 260 is a transverse section through the midabdomen with the solid mass seen anteriorly and the fluid in the dependent portions. Figure 261 is a transverse scan through the pelvis with fluid surrounding the uterus. We are easily able to identify the uterus in this case because of the linear echo arising from the endometrial cavity. It was originally felt to be a neoplastic tumor in the region of the solid mass with malignant ascites. At surgery, however, the patient was found to have a ruptured dermoid. Pathology revealed this to be a benign cystic teratoma with no evidence of malignancy. The ultrasound examination was extremely worrisome, for it suggested malignancy. The possibility

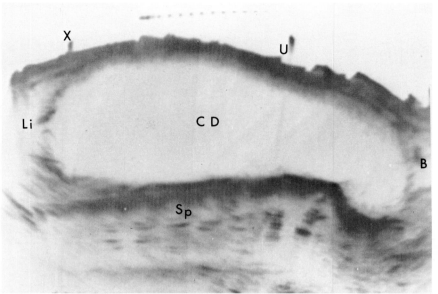

Fig. 258

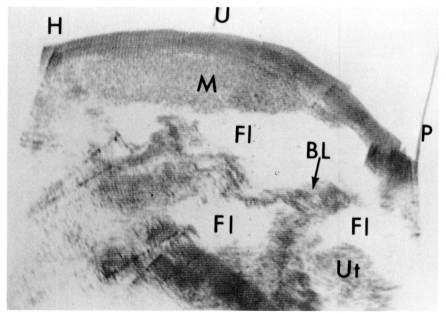

Fig. 259

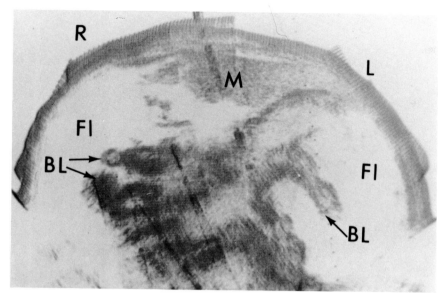

Fig. 260

of an ectopic pregnancy was also considered, since the anterior mass looked very much like placental tissue.

SOURCE: The case for figure 258 is provided through the courtesy of Dr. B. Green, M. D. Anderson Hospital, University of Texas Medical Center, Houston, Texas.

B	=	Urinary bladder
Bl	=	Bowel loops
CD	=	Cystic teratoma
EC	=	Endometrial cavity
Fl	=	Fluid in the abdomen
H	=	Head
L	=	Left
Li	=	Liver
M	=	Solid component to the ruptured dermoid
P	=	Level of the symphysis pubis
R	=	Right
Sp	=	Spine
U	=	Umbilical level
Ut	=	Uterus
X	=	Xyphoid level

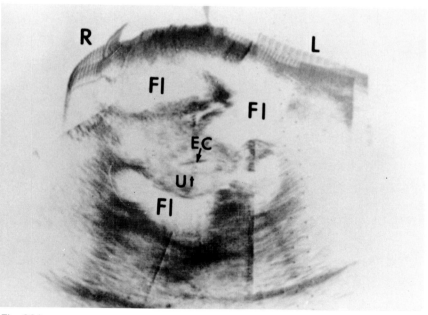

Fig. 261

Dermoids   II.

Figures 262 and 263 are scans of a patient with ultrasound examination for a pelvic and abdominal mass. The uterus is displaced posteriorly on the longitudinal scan (fig. 262). A mass is impinging on the urinary bladder. It has a mixed pattern to it, with a large fluid component. Numerous echogenic areas, however, are noted and indicate a solid mass. In figure 263 we see numerous curvilinear echoes (arrows) suggesting septations running through this mass. This also turned out to be a dermoid. Dermoids have numerous elements within them which yield a mixed ultrasonic echo pattern. The possibility of a septated ovarian cyst, cystadenoma, or cystadenocarcinoma could not be ruled out by the ultrasonic findings.

The scans in figures 264 and 265 were from a 23-year-old woman with a pelvic mass. In figure 264 we see the uterus displaced somewhat anteriorly by an extremely echogenic mass in the region of the cul-de-sac. The mass has somewhat ill-defined borders and is fairly difficult to see. It could be confused for bowel in the pelvis, except for the soft-echo appearance. Bowel usually is more echogenic. A pelvic X-ray (fig. 265) demonstrated a fat density in the pelvis. This indicated a dermoid. At surgery, a 13-cm, right ovarian mass was found which contained abundant sebum, hair, and a mixture of epidermis, dermal appendages, adipose tissue, and gastric mucosa. These echogenic dermoids usually contain a fair amount of hair and adipose tissue which yield high-level echoes on ultrasound.

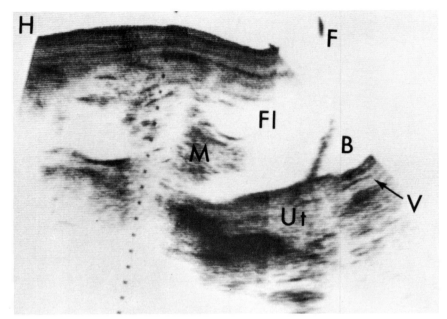

Fig. 262

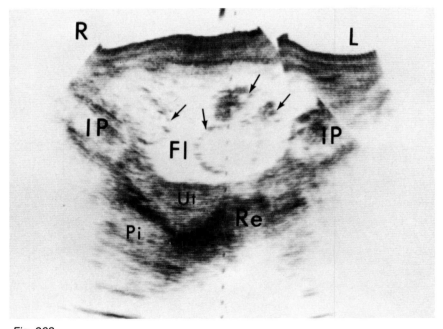

Fig. 263

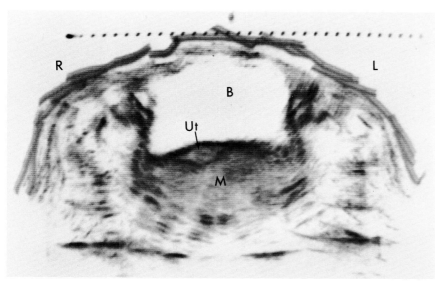

Fig. 264

Arrows = Curvilinear septa within the mass
B   = Urinary bladder
F   = Foot
Fl   = Fluid
H   = Head
IP   = Iliopsoas muscles
L   = Left
M   = Solid portion to the mass (fig. 262)
M   = Mass posterior to the uterus (fig. 264)
Pi   = Piriform muscle
R   = Right
Re   = Rectum
Ut   = Uterus
V   = Vagina

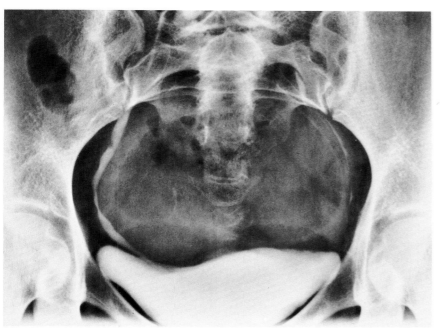

Fig. 265

Dermoids III.

One of the most difficult lesions to detect with ultrasound is an extremely echogenic dermoid. Frequently, dermoids with high-amplitude echoes will be missed during a pelvic ultrasound examination. This is because the high-amplitude echoes arising from the dermoids blend in with the surrounding high-amplitude echoes of the bowel and rectum in the pelvis. Certain clues, however, help in detecting these lesions. If the referring gynecologist describes a large mass in the adnexa, and no lesion can be identified, it is extremely important to look for an echogenic dermoid.

Figures 266 and 267 are scans of a patient with left adnexal mass palpated by the referring physician. A transverse scan (fig. 266) demonstrates the extremely important sign of bladder wall indentation (arrows); this gives a clue as to the site and size of the mass. Here we see an extremely echogenic dermoid in the left adnexa displacing the uterus to the right side. The size of the mass can be measured from the bladder wall (arrows) to the piriform muscle on the left side. The mass could have been missed easily, except for the bladder wall indentation. Figure 267 is a longitudinal scan of the mass seen just inferior to a normal portion of the ovary. At surgery, a 7-cm dermoid was found, and this contained a large amount of sebaceous material along with hair and some adipose tissue. Usually, the dermoids containing a large amount of hair are the ones which will yield high-level echoes that can be lost in the pelvis.

Figures 268 and 269 are of another patient who presented with a pelvic mass on the right side, as noted by physical examination. Again we see the important sign of indentation on the bladder wall (arrows), this time on the right side. An echogenic mass is situated between the bladder wall and piriform muscle on the right side. The normal left ovary is seen between the uterus and the piriform muscle on the left side. A longitudinal scan of the right adnexa demonstrates the bladder wall indentation and the high-amplitude echo of the mass. It is obvious how easily this

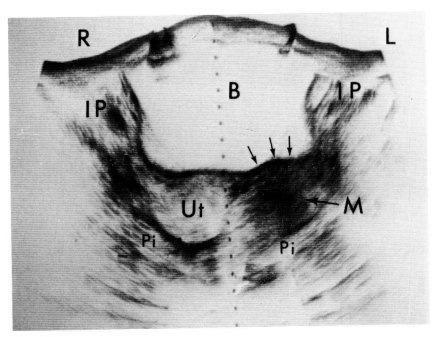

Fig. 266

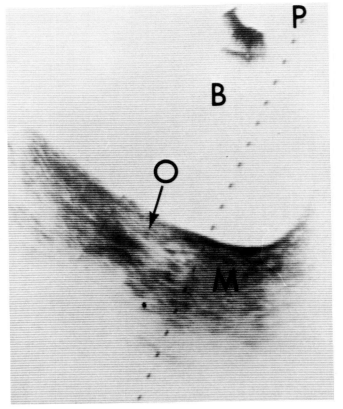

Fig. 267

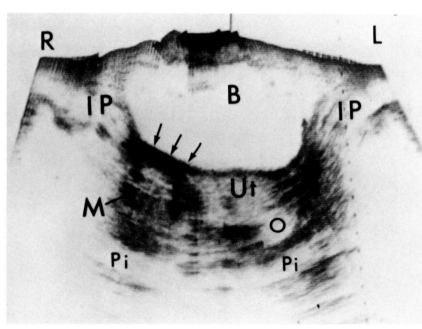

Fig. 268

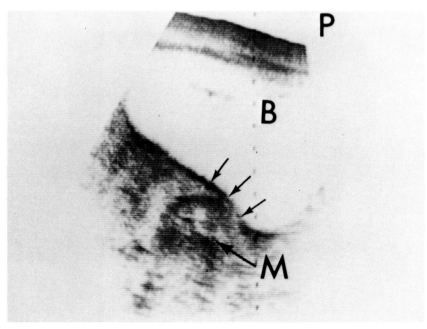

Fig. 269

mass might be lost in the high-amplitude echoes of the normal pelvis. If the referring physician states that there might be a large mass in the pelvis, we should be careful, for an echogenic dermoid could be missed on an ultrasound examination quite easily. It is extremely important to evaluate the contour of the bladder wall. This may provide the first clue that a mass is present. It is also extremely important to evaluate the high-amplitude echogenicity surrounding the uterus, ovaries, and normal pelvic musculature. If a region of echogenicity appears markedly different from the remainder of the pelvis, the possibility of an echogenic dermoid should be considered.

Arrows = Indentation on the bladder wall
B = Urinary bladder
IP = Iliopsoas muscle
L = Left
M = Echogenic dermoid
O = Ovary
P = Level of the symphysis pubis
Pi = Piriform muscle
R = Right
Ut = Uterus

Pelvic Inflammatory Disease   I.

Pelvic inflammatory disease presents an ultrasonic spectrum that depends upon the stage of infection. In an acute abscess, the masses within the pelvis will appear sonolucent and compatible with fluid. In a chronic abscess, however, the fibrosis and scarring will yield solid-appearing masses in the pelvis, which may be difficult to distinguish from neoplasms.

Figures 270 and 271 are of a 19-year-old young woman with a recent onset of pelvic pain. She was found clinically to have pelvic inflammatory disease and responded to antibiotics. Ultrasound examination demonstrated several fluid-filled areas in the right adnexal region compatible with tubal abscesses. The indentation on the urinary bladder wall indicating a right adnexal mass is notable. Fluid is seen in the tube as it loops over on itself in the right adenexa. The patient was found to have a positive gonococcal culture and responded well to antibiotic therapy.

Figures 272 and 273 are fairly characteristic pelvic scans of a patient with acute pelvic inflammatory disease. This 17-year-old girl had an onset of pelvic pain several weeks earlier. Pelvic ultrasound demonstrated fluid in the cul-de-sac. This sonolucent mass in the cul-de-sac does not appear to be as contained as we would see in an ovarian cyst or in an ovarian neoplasm. Rather, the fluid collection is noted in the cul-de-sac posterior to the uterus and filling the potential space of the lower peritoneal cavity. This was secondary to a collection of suppurative material in the cul-de-sac. The patient also responded well to antibiotics, leading to the diagnosis of pelvic inflammatory disease.

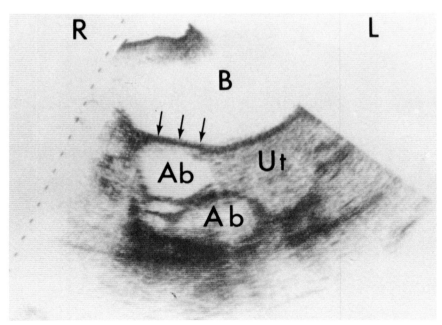

Fig. 270

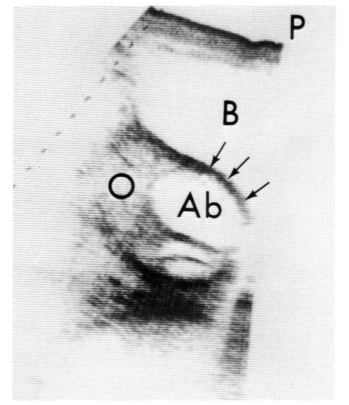

Fig. 271

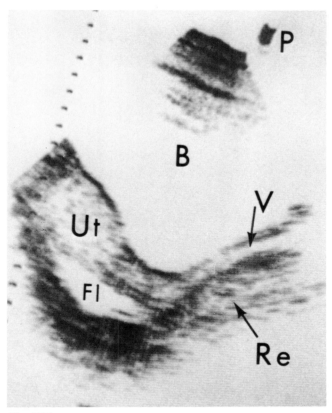

Fig. 272

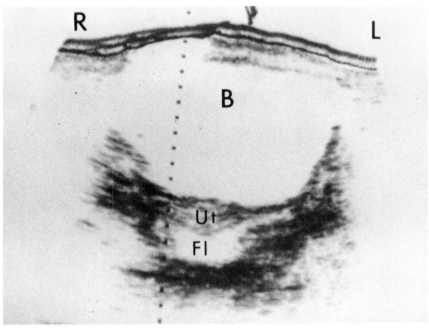

Fig. 273

Pelvic Inflammatory Disease II.

Pelvic inflammatory disease frequently is associated with an intrauterine device. Figure 274 is a longitudinal scan with a strong echo within the uterus, indicating an intrauterine device. This has a fairly characteristic appearance of a Copper 7 or a Copper T intrauterine device. Posterior to the uterus is a large sonolucent mass that is secondary to a cul-de-sac abscess. Here we see a somewhat irregular border to this sonolucent mass, highly consistent with an abscess. The possibility of a hematoma could not be ruled out. Clinically, however, the finding was consistent with pelvic inflammatory disease.

Often, long-standing pelvic inflammatory disease leads to hydrosalpinx. This entity is actually a sterile collection that has been scarred and blocked within the fallopian tube. The sonolucent collection in the fallopian tube often gives a picture similar to an ovarian cyst.

Figure 275 is an example of a moderately sized hydrosalpinx in the right fallopian tube. Again we see indentation on the posterior bladder wall characteristic of a right adnexal lesion. The hydrosalpinx is extremely lucent, indicating its fluid-filled nature. The walls are fairly sharp, although not quite as sharp as we might see in a simple ovarian cyst.

Figures 276 and 277 represent a hydrosalpinx that is somewhat larger than the one in figure 275. The walls of this hydrosalpinx are slightly sharper than in the previous case. This one could be confused with an ovarian cyst, or possibly a cystadenoma.

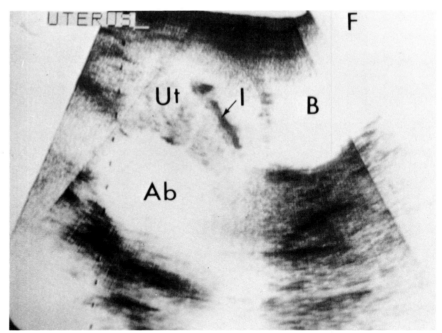

Fig. 274

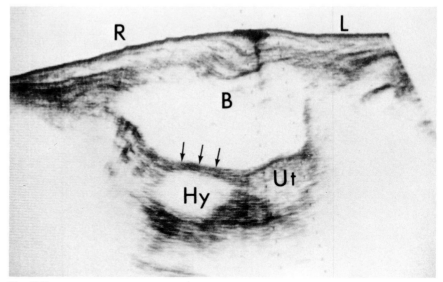

Fig. 275

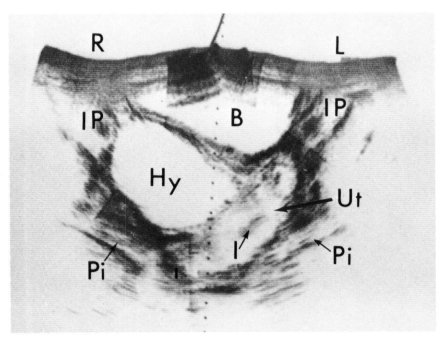

Fig. 276

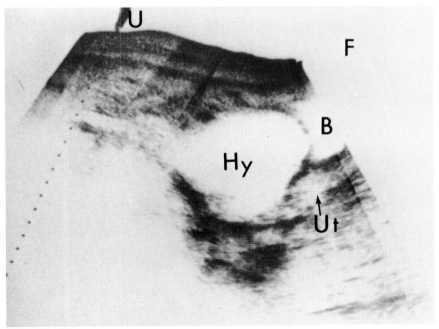

Fig. 277

Ab   = Cul-de-sac abscess
Arrows = Indentation on the bladder wall
B   = Urinary bladder
F   = Foot
Hy   = Hydrosalpinx
I   = Intrauterine device
IP   = Iliopsoas muscle
L   = Left
Pi   = Piriform muscle
R   = Right
U   = Umbilical level
Ut   = Uterus

Pelvic Inflammatory Disease III.

Pelvic inflammatory disease also can appear to have a mixed echo pattern, rather than just a sonolucent echo pattern. Usually, when a mixed echo pattern of solid and cystic lesions is present, it is more characteristic of an abscess as is found elsewhere in the body.

Figures 278 and 279 are of a patient with severe pelvic inflammatory disease associated with an abscess anterior to the uterus and thickening of the urinary bladder wall. There also is evidence of debris (arrows) within the urinary bladder itself. The relatively sonolucent collection between the uterus and bladder wall has an appearance more characteristic of an abscess. Irregular borders are demonstrated. The internal echoes arising from the abscess also have an appearance of debris rather than a solid nature. There is evidence of some through transmission through the abscess; again, this is somewhat characteristic.

Figures 280 and 281 are scans of a 21-year-old woman who had an intrauterine device removed 1 day previously because of pelvic pain. An ultrasound examination demonstrated two relatively lucent areas in the pelvis. It was difficult to visualize the uterus. Figure 280 is a transverse scan demonstrating the uterus in the mid pelvis. The borders of the uterus (arrows), however, are quite difficult to see because of the adherent adnexal masses. Bilateral abscesses are present. Because of the inflammatory reaction, the interface between the abscesses and the uterus may be quite difficult to see. The abscesses present with a mixed echo pattern in which a portion is relatively sonolucent, indicating suppurative material, and a portion is echogenic, indicating fibrosis and debris. Figure 281 is a longitudinal scan of the patient with the abscess collection posterior to the uterus.

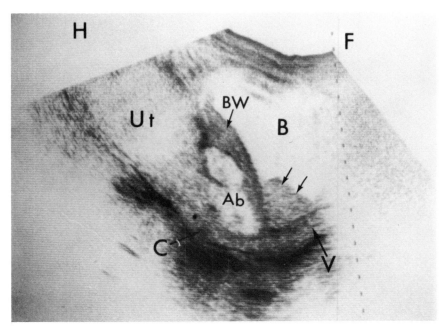

Fig. 278

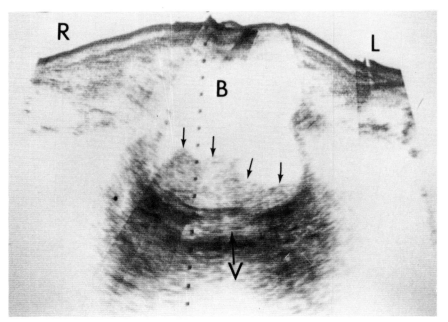

Fig. 279

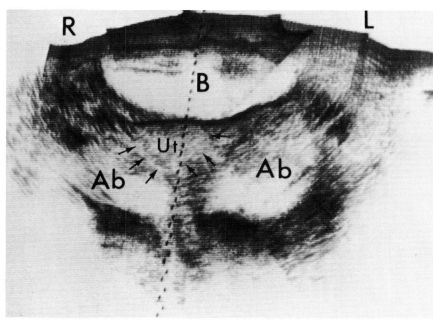

Fig. 280

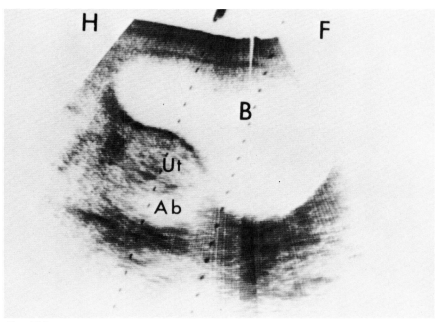

Fig. 281

Ab	= Pelvic abscess
Arrows	= Debris in the urinary bladder wall
B	= Urinary bladder
BW	= Thickened urinary bladder wall
C	= Cervix
F	= Foot
H	= Head
L	= Left
R	= Right
Ut	= Uterus
Ut and arrows	= Uterus that is difficult to see secondary to surrounding abscess
V	= Vagina

Pelvic Inflammatory Disease IV.

Occasionally, pelvic inflammatory disease can be so echogenic that a solid lesion of the pelvis may be diagnosed by ultrasound. Whenever a chronic abscess is present, the interfaces between the uterus and adnexa are difficult to distinguish with ultrasound due to the loss of an acoustic plane. Often a fibroid uterus or uterine tumor is considered when chronic pelvic inflammatory disease is present. The other possibility is an ovarian neoplasm.

Figure 282 is a transverse scan of a large pelvic mass. It is difficult to distinguish this from the uterus. A slight border, however, can be defined on the right side (small arrows). It is difficult to see because of the adherent abscess. Again we see indentation on the urinary bladder (large arrow) secondary to the right adnexal mass. This large abscess could be considered a solid ovarian tumor. Some through transmission is suggested, however, and this often can lead to the diagnosis of an abscess. It is important to have clinical information confirming the diagnosis of pelvic inflammatory disease.

In figure 283, a transverse scan, again it is difficult to see the uterus. There is the slight suggestion of a border to the uterus (arrows), but this is difficult to see because of the echogenic mass. This left mass was secondary to a chronic abscess in which the border to the uterus was lost because of inflammatory adhesions.

Figure 284 is an example of a right adnexal abscess that is more easily separated from the uterus. An interface between the uterus and the right adnexa actually can be seen, but the echogenicity and size of this abscess would be extremely worrisome for an ovarian neoplasm. Abscesses present a spectrum from fluid-filled to mixed to solid-appearing lesions in the pelvis. They can be confused for several other entities. Clinical correlation is extremely important in coming to the correct diagnosis.

Figure 285 shows an interesting case of pelvic inflammatory disease, which at first sight, could be confused

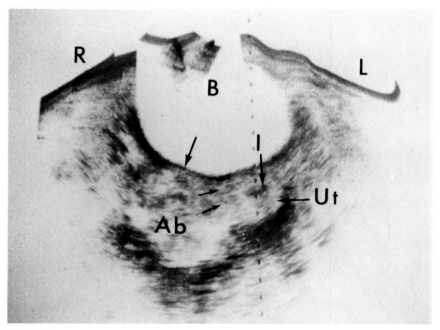

Fig. 282

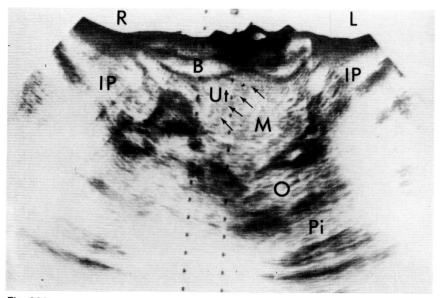

Fig. 283

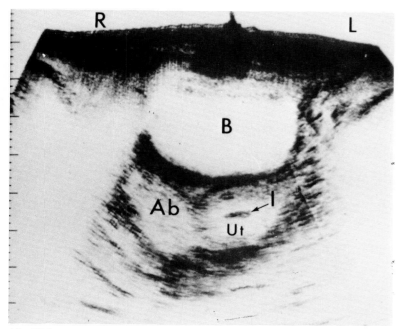

Fig. 284

for an ectopic pregnancy. Here we see a suggestion of a circular gestational sac. Surrounding this sac is a relatively sonolucent mass (arrows) which turned out to be a chronic abscess secondary to pelvic inflammatory disease.

SOURCE: The case in figure 285 is provided through the courtesy of Dr. F. Taber, Valley Presbyterian Hospital, Van Nuys, California.

Ab	= Pelvic abscess
B	= Urinary bladder
C	= Cervix
?gs	= Pelvic inflammatory disease suggesting an ectopic pregnancy
H	= Head
I	= Intrauterine device
IP	= Iliopsoas muscle
Large arrow	= Indentation on the urinary bladder
L	= Left
M	= Pelvic abscess
O	= Ovary
P	= Level of the symphysis pubis
Pi	= Piriform muscle
R	= Right
Small arrows	= Uterine interface
Ut	= Uterus
V	= Vagina

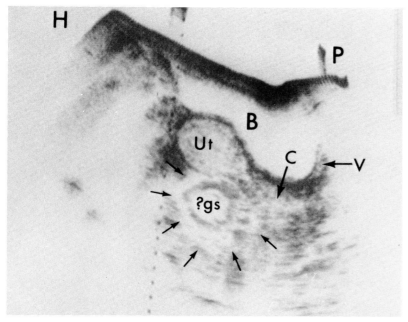

Fig. 285

Endometriosis   I.

Endometriosis can be the great mimicker in pelvic ultrasound evaluation, similar to pelvic inflammatory disease. Just as in pelvic inflammatory disease, endometriosis can give a spectrum of ultrasonic appearances, ranging from a nearly completely sonolucent mass all the way to a highly echogenic solid. Figures 286–288 are of a patient with a large pelvic mass secondary to endometriosis. The large cephalic sonolucent portion of the mass is a fluid-filled endometrioma. A solid component to the endometriosis, however, is posterior to the uterus. The greater echogenicity of this region in the cul-de-sac is most likely due to clotted blood, debris, or fibrosis. A transverse scan of the same patient (fig. 288) demonstrates the endometrioma with soft echoes within it, just posterior and to the left of the uterus.

Figure 289 is of another patient with a large fluid-filled endometrioma in the left adnexa. The left adnexal mass is impinging on the posterior urinary bladder wall (arrows) as noted earlier. The endometrioma is displacing the left ovary away from the uterus. The ultrasonic findings of this endometrioma would not be specific for this entity. Other possibilities would include an abscess, an ovarian cyst, or possibly cystadenoma.

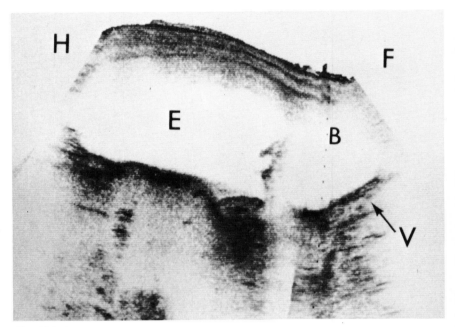

Fig. 286

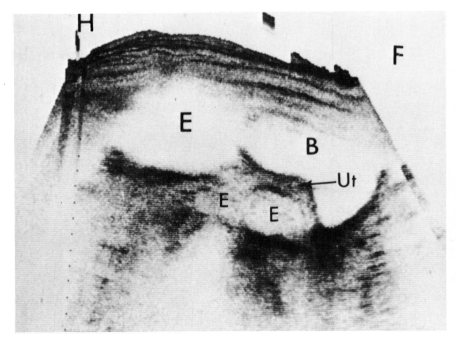

Fig. 287

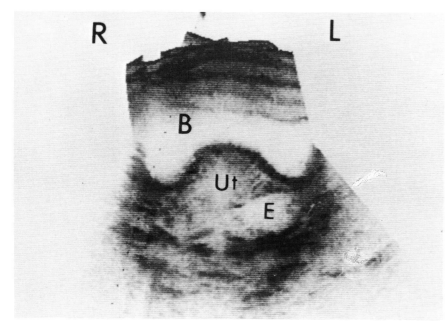

Fig. 288

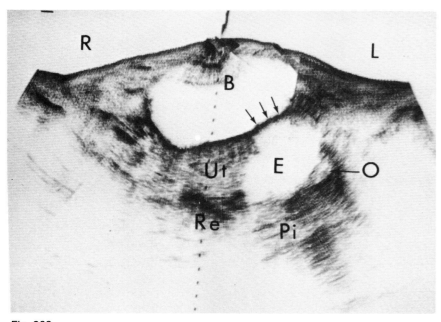

Fig. 289

Arrows	=	Indentation of the endometrioma on the bladder wall
B	=	Urinary bladder
E	=	Endometriosis
F	=	Foot
H	=	Head
L	=	Left
O	=	Left ovary
Pi	=	Piriform muscle
R	=	Right
Re	=	Rectum
Ut	=	Uterus
V	=	Vagina

Endometriosis   II.

Figure 290 is a pelvic ultrasound scan of a 25-year-old woman with a large pelvic mass. The ultrasound demonstrated a large mixed mass superior to the uterus, which eventually was found to be an endometrioma. Within the sonolucent endometrioma are numerous echoes secondary to debris. Also present is a cul-de-sac endometrioma posterior to the uterus. This is an example of an endometrioma with a mixed echo pattern. It could not be distinguished from an abscess or an ovarian lesion.

Figures 291 and 292 are scans of a 34-year-old woman with carcinoma of the breast. She was noted to have pelvic masses on physical examination, and an ultrasound examination was performed. Here we see several large masses in the cul-de-sac and right adnexa. The mass in the cul-de-sac is solid in nature, and the interface between this mass and the uterus is quite difficult to see. The right adnexal mass has a sonolucent central fluid collection. With the patient's history, the possibility of ovarian neoplasm was considered quite likely. At surgery, however, she was found to have bilateral ovarian chocolate hemorrhagic cysts which indicated endometriosis rather than ovarian neoplasm. This case illustrates the marked difficulty in dealing with the ultrasonic findings of endometriosis. Because of its similarity to pelvic inflammatory disease, this entity can present as a spectrum of findings which can be confused with other pelvic pathology.

Figure 293 is another example of endometriosis with a very solid-appearing mass in the right adnexa, displacing the uterus to the left side. Again the possibility of a solid ovarian neoplasm could not be ruled out. This mass also could be consistent with a chronic abscess.

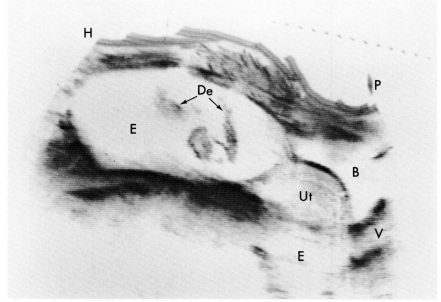

Fig. 290

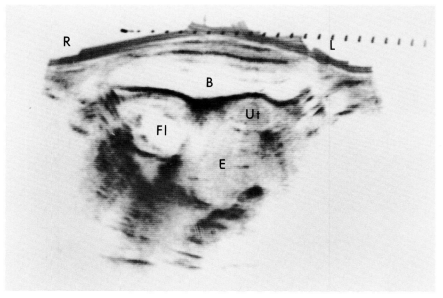

Fig. 291

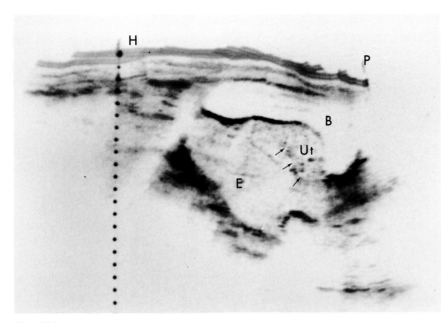

Fig. 292

SOURCE: The cases in figures 290–292 are provided through the courtesy of Dr. B. Green, M. D. Anderson Hospital, University of Texas Medical Center, Houston, Texas.

Arrows = Separation between uterus and endometrioma
B = Urinary bladder
De = Debris
E = Endometrioma
Fl = Fluid in the endometrioma
H = Head
I = Intrauterine device
IP = Iliopsoas muscle
L = Left
P = Level of the pelvis
R = Right
Ut = Uterus
V = Vagina

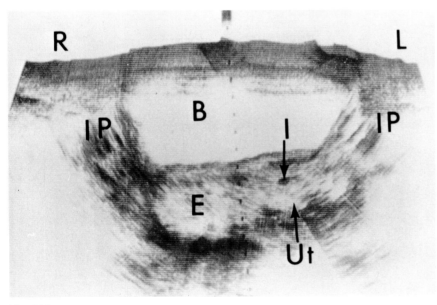

Fig. 293

Endometriosis III.

Figures 294 and 295 demonstrate a solid-appearing endometrioma in the right adnexa. The urinary bladder wall is indented, indicating a right adnexal mass. Although this endometrioma appears solid in nature, there is evidence of fluid in the cul-de-sac. The patient underwent surgery, and a large endometrioma involving the right ovary and posterior uterine wall was found.

Figures 296 and 297 are scans of a 26-year-old woman who entered the hospital complaining of lower-abdominal pain. Her abdominal pain started at age 18 and was associated with dysmenorrhea. The dysmenorrhea, however, disappeared when she was placed on oral contraceptives. In the preceding year the symptoms became worse, and she finally entered the hospital because of increasing abdominal pain associated with her menstruation. A pelvic ultrasound examination was performed (figs. 296 and 297). The transverse scan (fig. 296) demonstrates the uterus surrounded by a large echogenic mass. The interesting point in this case is that the mass penetrates the urinary bladder wall (arrows). The longitudinal scan demonstrates the uterus to be somewhat retroverted. The large endometrioma is difficult to separate from the fundus of the uterus. Again we see invasion of the urinary wall by this echogenic mass. At surgery, this patient was found to have an endometrioma involving the fundal portion of the uterus and posterosuperior aspect of the bladder wall. This portion of the urinary bladder had to be resected. Pathological examination demonstrated the urinary bladder wall to be involved with endometriosis. Ultrasound examination was extremely helpful in delineating the extent and nature of this disease.

It must be remembered that endometriosis can be situated any place in the abdomen. In this case, the finding of bladder wall thickening could not be distinguished from a bladder wall tumor. With the clinical history, however, the diagnosis of endometriosis was most likely.

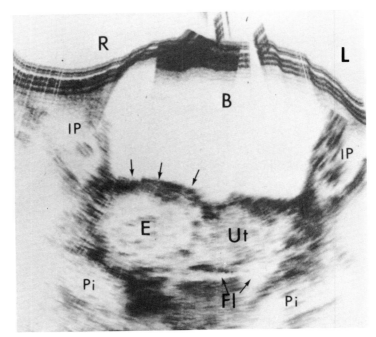

Fig. 294

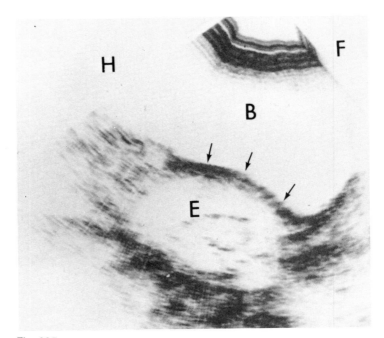

Fig. 295

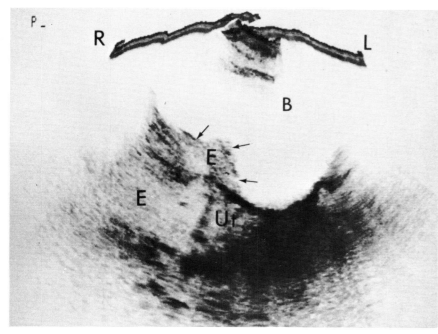

Fig. 296

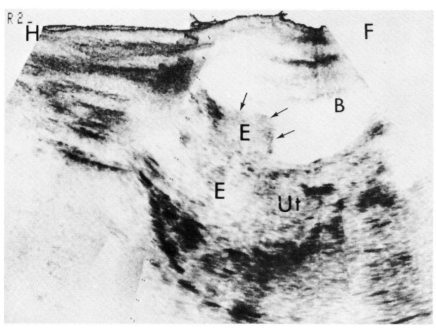

Fig. 297

Arrows	=	Indentation on urinary bladder wall (figs. 294 and 295)
Arrows	=	Urinary bladder wall invaded by endometriosis (figs. 296 and 297)
B	=	Urinary bladder
E	=	Endometrioma
F	=	Foot
Fl	=	Fluid
H	=	Head
IP	=	Iliopsoas muscle
L	=	Left
Pi	=	Piriform muscle
R	=	Right
Ut	=	Uterus

Pelvic Lymphadenopathy

Figures 298 and 299 are pelvic scans
obtained from a patient with stage III
Hodgkin's disease. In the pelvis, as elsewhere in the body, lymphadenopathy
presents as relatively sonolucent
masses. The transverse scan (fig. 298)
demonstrates the lymph nodes indenting
the lateral superior aspect of the urinary
bladder on the right side.

Figure 299 is a longitudinal scan
of lymph node enlargement in the pelvis
and lower abdomen. The characteristic
feature of lymphadenopathy is usually
a sonolucent mass with no marked enhanced through transmission. Such
masses, however, are so sonolucent
that they may be confused for cystic
lesions.

SOURCE: The cases in figures 298 and 299
are provided through the courtesy of Dr.
B. Green, M. D. Anderson Hospital, University of Texas Medical Center, Houston,
Texas.

B = Urinary bladder
L = Left
M = Marked lymph node enlargement
P = Level of the symphysis pubis
R = Right
U = Level of the umbilicus

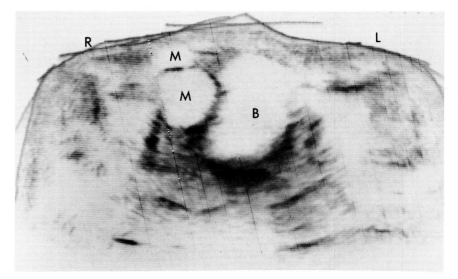

Fig. 298

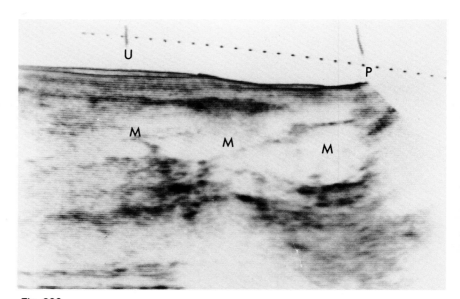

Fig. 299

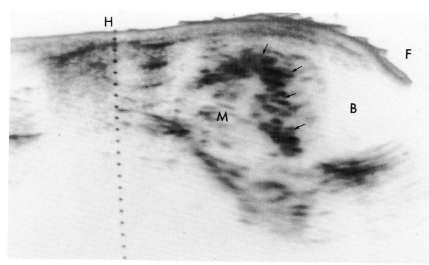

Fig. 300

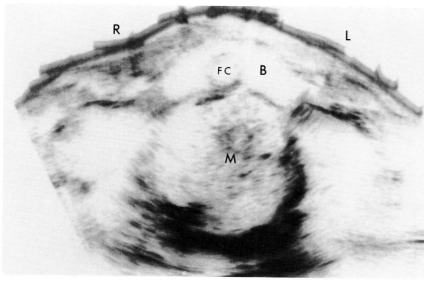

Fig. 301

Adenocarcinoma of the Colon; Liposarcoma

Figure 300 is a longitudinal scan of a woman with diffuse metastatic colonic carcinoma throughout the pelvis. A large mass is seen posterior to the urinary bladder. A portion of the mass is highly echogenic (arrows). Mucinous colonic carcinomas often give a high-amplitude echo. This patient had diffuse pelvic metastasis which impinged on the urinary bladder only slightly.

Figure 301 is a transverse scan of an elderly patient with recurrent pelvic liposarcoma. A large mass is seen posterior to the urinary bladder. There is no characteristic finding suggesting the etiology of this tumor. A Foley catheter is seen in place within the urinary bladder. This mass was found to be diffuse liposarcoma of the pelvis.

SOURCE: The cases in figures 300 and 301 were provided through the courtesy of Dr. B. Green, M. D. Anderson Hospital, Texas University Medical Center, Houston, Texas.

Arrows	=	Highly echogenic regions in a mucinous adenocarcinoma of the colon
B	=	Urinary bladder
F	=	Foot
FC	=	Foley catheter
H	=	Head
L	=	Left
M	=	Solid pelvic masses
R	=	Right

Bladder Duplication Artifacts: Foley Catheter; Blood Clot; Vaginal Carcinoma

Figure 302 is an excellent example of a bladder duplication artifact. It has already been mentioned that a bladder can often present as a sonolucent mass in the pelvis, secondary to a duplication artifact. In this instance, we have a complete duplication artifact of the bladder that is situated posterior to the urinary bladder. What makes this scan so interesting is the duplication artifact of the vagina. The vaginal duplication artifact is situated posterior to the duplication artifact of the bladder. The artifact arises from the strong echo off the posterior urinary bladder wall hitting the transducer-skin interface and making a second trip. This yields a duplication artifact of the urinary bladder and the vagina. Duplication artifacts are discussed in greater detail elsewhere in this volume.

Figure 303 illustrates a mass secondary to a Foley catheter within the urinary bladder. This is quite easy to detect once it is recognized. The distal portion of the tube extending from the water-filled portion of the Foley catheter also is seen.

Figure 304 is a transverse scan of the urinary bladder with an echogenic mass on the posterior wall. Although this could represent a bladder tumor, it is a blood clot which presented as an echogenic mass within the urinary bladder.

Figure 305 is a longitudinal scan of a patient who had a hysterectomy 15 years previously. She was found to have a mass posterior to the urinary bladder on ultrasound examination. The lucent anterior portion of the vagina is seen directly posterior to the urinary bladder. Deep to this, however, is an echogenic mass which turned out to be a vaginal tumor. This vaginal carcinoma would be somewhat difficult to separate from the rectum as far as ultrasound is concerned. We see the lucent anterior muscularis of the vagina, however, separated from the vaginal tumor by a strong echogenic interface. The strong echogenic interface represents the vaginal mucosa. This unusual case

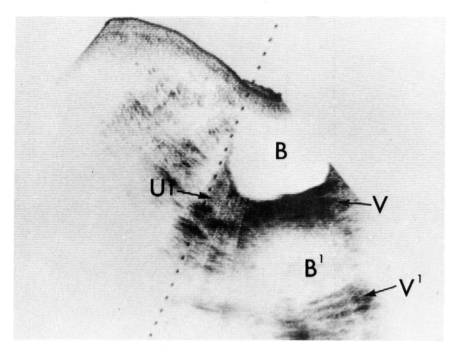

Fig. 302

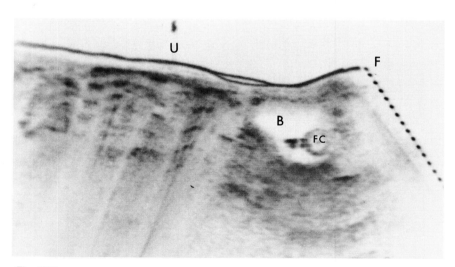

Fig. 303

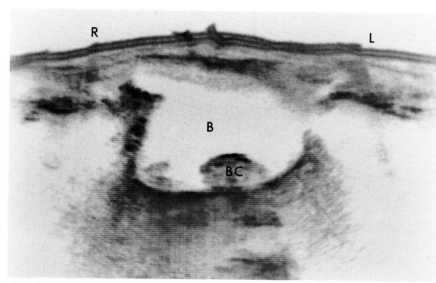

Fig. 304

demonstrates the marked thickening of the muscularis region of the posterior aspect of the vagina as compared to the relatively normal thickness for the anterior vaginal muscular area.

SOURCE: Figures 303 and 304 are provided through the courtesy of Dr. B. Green, M. D. Anderson Hospital, Texas Medical Center, Houston, Texas.

B	=	Urinary bladder
BC	=	Blood clot
B¹	=	Bladder duplication artifact
F	=	Foot
FC	=	Foley catheter
L	=	Left
P	=	Level of the symphysis pubis
R	=	Right
T	=	Vaginal tumor
U	=	Umbilical level
Ut	=	Uterus
V	=	Normal vaginal region anteriorly
V	=	Vagina
V¹	=	Vaginal duplication artifact
Vm	=	Vaginal mucosa
VT	=	Vaginal tumor

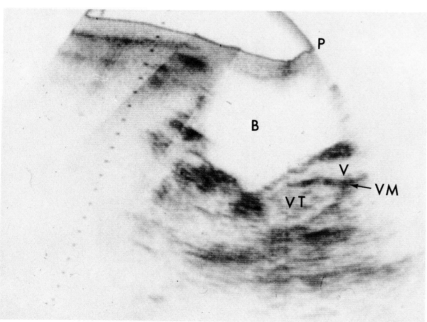

Fig. 305

Bladder Tumors

Figures 306 and 307 are pelvic scans of a 42-year-old woman who had some difficulty on urination. The longitudinal scan (fig. 306) demonstrates bladder wall thickening (arrows) on the posterior aspect. The bladder wall is approximately 1–1.5 cm in thickness, directly anterior to the vagina. Figure 307 is a transverse scan of the bladder wall thickening (arrows) on the posterior aspect of the bladder. The soft echoes, with no evidence of shadowing, indicate a soft-tissue tumor. This could represent either a blood clot or debris in the bladder. With the suggestion of wall thickening, however, a bladder tumor is most likely. At surgery, the patient was found to have urinary bladder carcinoma on the posterior left aspect of the bladder wall.

Another example of a urinary bladder wall carcinoma is seen in figures 308 and 309. The bladder tumor is approximately 2 cm in thickness. We see a marked irregular surface to the bladder wall which is in contact with urine (arrows). Also noted on the transverse scan in figure 308 is a circular structure secondary to a Foley catheter. When a soft tissue density is noted within the urinary bladder or urinary bladder wall, the possibility of a urinary bladder carcinoma should be considered.

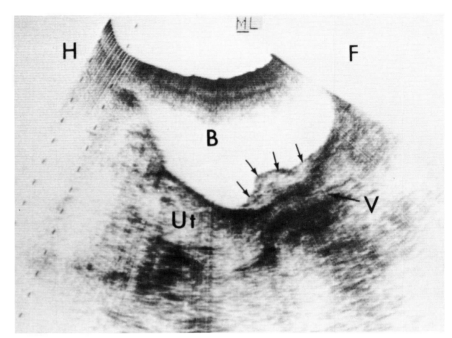

Fig. 306

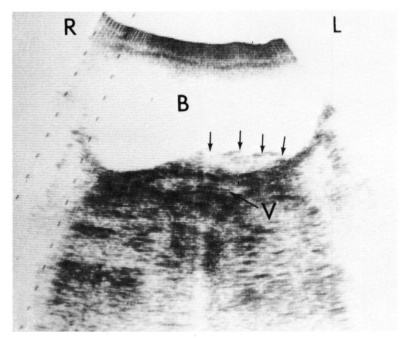

Fig. 307

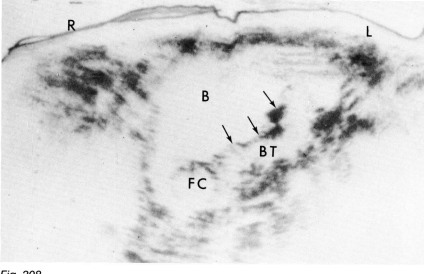

Arrows = Urinary bladder wall carcinoma
B   = Urinary bladder
BT   = Urinary bladder wall tumor
F   = Foot
FC   = Foley catheter
H   = Head
L   = Left
R   = Right
Ut   = Uterus
V   = Vagina

Fig. 308

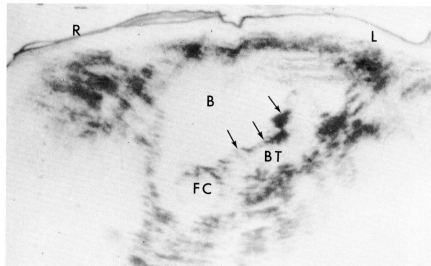

Fig. 309

Urinary Bladder Diverticulum

Figure 310 is a longitudinal scan of the pelvis with a sonolucent mass posterior to the urinary bladder. This may be considered an ovarian cyst or other fluid-filled structure. The possibility of a bladder diverticulum, however, should be considered. In figure 310 the communication between the urinary bladder and the bladder diverticulum is not demonstrated. Figures 311 and 312 of the same patient do, however, demonstrate communication in the longitudinal and transverse planes. We see an opening, approximately 6–7 mm in diameter, indicating the communication between the bladder and the bladder diverticulum. If this communication can be seen, the diagnosis and explanation of the sonolucent mass can be determined.

Figure 313 is another example of a bladder diverticulum in the right pelvis, lateral to the urinary bladder.

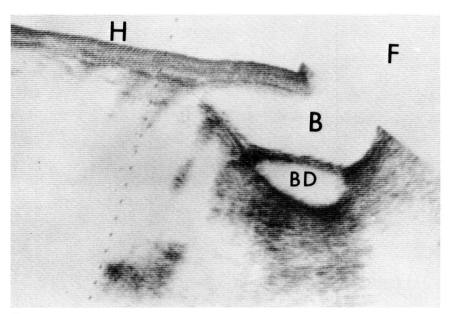

Fig. 310

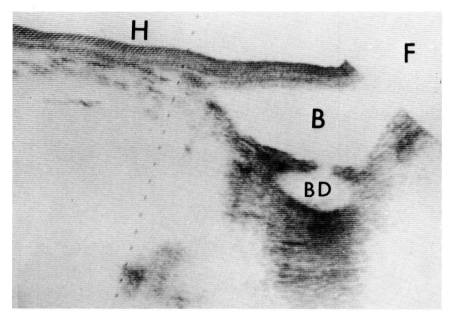

Fig. 311

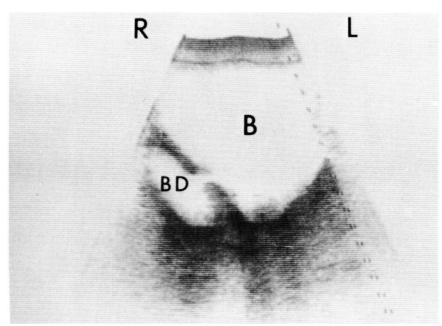

Fig. 312

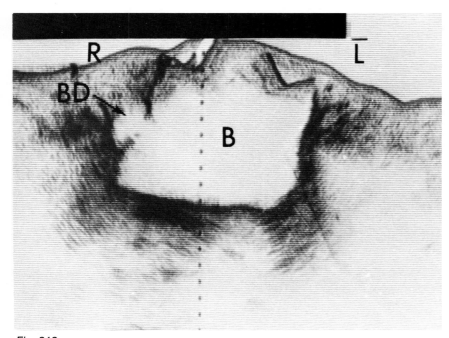

Fig. 313

B = Urinary bladder
BD = Bladder diverticulum
F = Foot
H = Head
L = Left
R = Right

Normal Prepubescent Pelvis

When examining the prepubescent pelvis, it is important to visualize the uterus in its long axis. Normally, the cervical region of the prepubescent uterus is larger than the fundal region.

Figures 314 and 315 are longitudinal scans of a female child approximately 4 years of age (fig. 314) and a female infant, 6 months of age (fig. 315). The cervical region is as large or larger than the fundal region in both cases. Following puberty and hormonal stimulation, a reversal will occur, and the fundus of the uterus will become larger and more bulbous than the cervical region. Examination of the newborn and the pediatric pelvis can be quite difficult because the patients move about quite markedly during the course of a study. It is important, however, to attempt to visualize the uterus. Real-time examination can often facilitate the study and yield more rapid examination.

Finding the ovaries in a prepubescent child is also difficult. They are usually quite small, 1 cm or less. Again, the study can be quite difficult but usually does not require anesthesia.

Figure 316 is a transverse scan demonstrating the ovaries bilaterally. The right ovary is approximately 1 cm in diameter, and the left ovary is less than 1 cm in diameter. Here we visualize the ovaries cephalad to the uterus. The rectum is seen between the ovaries.

Figure 317 is a longitudinal scan of the right ovary. It appears as a relatively sonolucent oval-shaped structure in the adnexa. The marked difficulty encountered in visualizing the ovaries is due to their small size and poor patient cooperation.

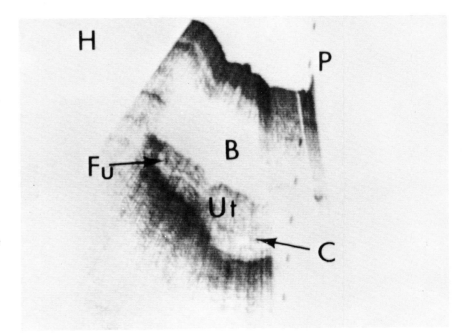

Fig. 314

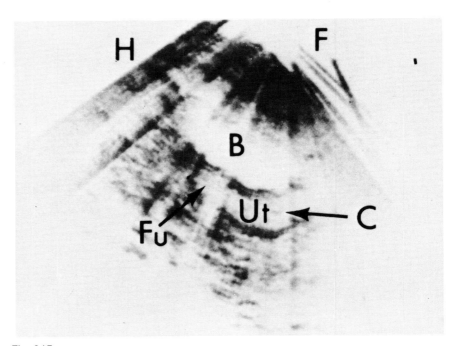

Fig. 315

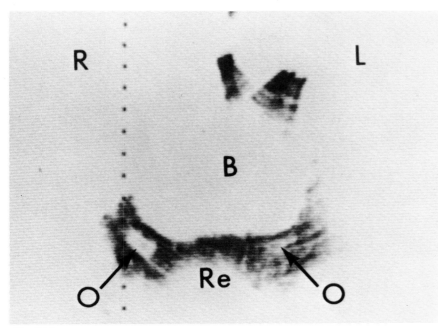

Fig. 316

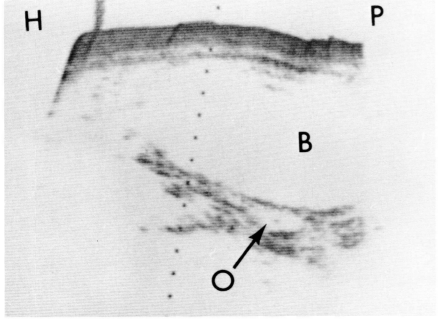

Fig. 317

B	=	Urinary bladder
C	=	Cervix
Fu	=	Fundus of the uterus
H	=	Head
L	=	Left
O	=	Ovaries
P	=	Level of the symphysis pubis
R	=	Right
Re	=	Rectum
Ut	=	Uterus

Precocious Puberty; Testicular Feminization

Figures 318–320 are scans of a 6-year-old child with precocious puberty. In precocious puberty, hormonal stimulation leads to changes in the uterus. The fundal size of the uterus is increased and becomes larger than the cervix. In a transverse scan (fig. 318) the uterus is visualized slightly to the left of midline. This uterus is much larger than normal in a 6-year-old. The ovaries are also quite large, measuring approximately 2 cm or greater in diameter in the transverse plane. Figure 319 is a longitudinal scan with a configuration of the uterus that is more characteristic of the adult, or poststimulated, uterus. The fundus has a more bulky or bulbous appearance than the cervical region. Usually, in the unstimulated uterus the fundus is much smaller than the cervical region. In this 6-year-old with precocious puberty, however, the fundus was large compared with the cervical region. Figure 320 is a longitudinal scan of the right ovary. Again, the ovary appears much larger than expected in a 6-year-old. Normally, this should be 1 cm or less in diameter. This ovary is at least 2 cm in diameter and is impinging on the posterior aspect of the urinary bladder.

Figure 321 is a transverse scan of a 16-year-old who entered the hospital for an evaluation of primary amenorhea. No pelvic organs can be seen. The uterus was not identified. Various pelvic musculature, such as the iliopsoas muscle, the obturator internus muscle, and the piriform muscles can be seen, but we were never able to identify the ovaries during the course of the examination. The patient also underwent a pelvic examination, and her vagina was found to end in a blind pouch. The cervix was not identified. The findings are consistent with testicular feminization. For this entity, a pelvic ultrasound can be quite helpful. We were looking for a normal prepubescent uterus and ovaries but were unable to identify any such structures during the course of pelvic sonography.

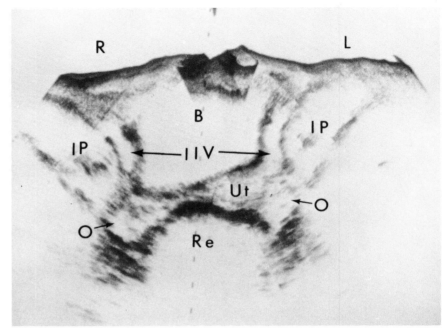

Fig. 318

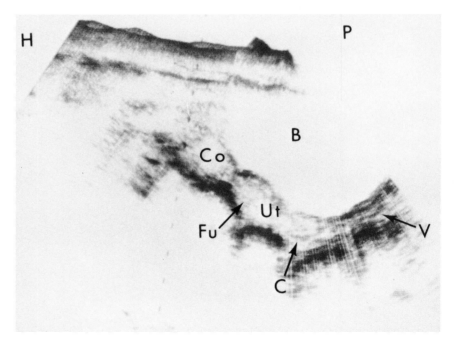

Fig. 319

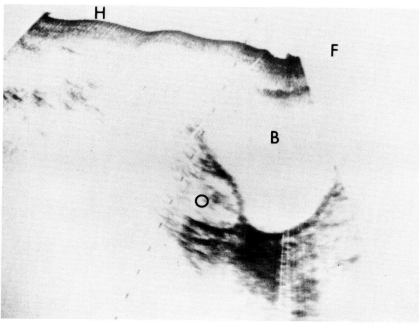

Fig. 320

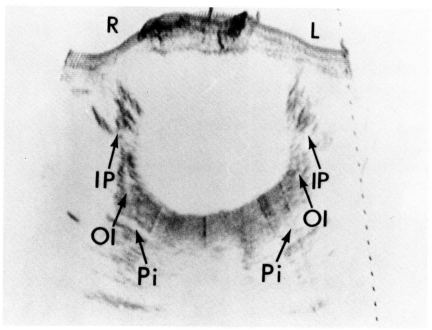

Fig. 321

B	=	Urinary bladder
C	=	Cervix
Co	=	Colon
F	=	Foot
Fu	=	Fundus of the uterus
H	=	Head
IIV	=	Internal iliac vessels
IP	=	Iliopsoas muscles
L	=	Left
O	=	Ovaries
OI	=	Obturator internus muscle
P	=	Level of the symphysis pubis
Pi	=	Piriform muscle
R	=	Right
Re	=	Rectum
Ut	=	Uterus
V	=	Vagina

Appendix: Ultrasound Physics and Technique

This section reviews the physics and technique of ultrasonography applied during ultrasound examinations. Production of a useful scan requires an adequate understanding of the concepts involved.

Piezoelectric Effect

The main component of all ultrasound systems is the piezoelectric crystal in the transducer. This crystal has the ability to change one form of energy into another. When a piezoelectric crystal is compressed by pressure, as by an echo returning from inside the patient, a voltage is generated across the two sides of the crystal. This is termed the *piezoelectric effect*. The reverse also occurs. When a voltage is applied across the crystal, it will expand and give off a pulse of ultrasound that will be transmitted into the patient. This is termed the *reverse piezoelectric effect*. Because of these properties, an ultrasound transducer acts both as transmitter and receiver when the pulse echo technique is applied.

The Pulse Echo Technique

When a voltage is applied across a piezoelectric crystal over a short period, the crystal expands rapidly and transmits a pulse of ultrasound into the patient. The crystal rings at its resonant frequency for 1 to 3 μsec and is dampened quickly. It is during this period, less than 1% of the application time, that the transducer is acting as a transmitter of ultrasound. The remainder of the time the transducer is waiting for the echoes that arise from inside the patient to return and strike the surface of the transducer. This waiting period is about 1 msec. During this time, the transducer is acting as a receiver. The returning echoes act as a pressure wave to compress the surface of the transducer. When a piezoelectric crystal is compressed, a voltage is given off by the crystal that is proportional to the strength of the returning echo.

This sequence of events is called the *pulse echo technique*. The crystal acts as a transmitter for a short period of time (1 to 3 μsec) and a receiver for a much longer period of time (approximately 1 to 2 msec). Depending on the unit in use, there are roughly 500 pulses per second accompanied by 500 listening periods.

Resonant Frequency

A wine glass struck with a spoon emits a pitch determined by the thickness of the glass. It will ring at its resonant frequency. The same thing happens to a piezoelectric crystal when it has a voltage quickly applied to its surfaces: it rings at a resonant frequency determined by its thickness. A crystal is constructed in such a manner that its thickness is half the wavelength (λ) of the resonant frequency. Therefore, the thickness of a piezoelectric crystal will determine the frequency of sound transmitted into the patient.

Interaction of Ultrasound with Body Tissue

Certain formulas are essential to an understanding of ultrasound reflection at different interfaces. The first basic formula illustrates the relation of velocity, frequency, and wavelength:

$$V = f\lambda. \tag{1}$$

The velocity of sound in tissue varies according to the density and elasticity of the tissue involved. Since for most soft tissues of the body the velocity is very similar, ultrasound units are constructed assuming a constant velocity of 1540 m/sec in soft tissue. Most soft tissue is close to this assumed velocity, with only slight variation. Structures composed of bone and air have a velocity dramatically different than the assumed velocity of 1540 m/sec. These create severe difficulties in diagnostic ultrasound and are discussed in the next section.

Equation (1) states that with a constant velocity an increase in frequency will necessitate a decrease in wavelength (λ), or vice versa. Remember that a piezoelectric crystal is constructed so that a thickness of $\lambda/2$ will determine its resonant frequency. Therefore, a thicker crystal (larger $\lambda/2$) corresponds to a lower frequency. A thinner crystal (smaller $\lambda/2$) will result in a higher-frequency transducer.

Acoustic Impedance and Reflection

Even though most soft tissue structures conduct sound at velocities close to 1540 m/sec, there is slight variation. This variation is the result of acoustic impedance, which may be expressed as

$$Z = V\rho, \tag{2}$$

where Z is acoustic impedance, V is velocity, and ρ is the density of tissue.

Acoustic impedance plays a major role in the amount of sound reflected at an interface of two substances in contact with each other. Remember that diagnostic ultrasound uses the pulse echo technique. The piezoelectric crystal is excited by a voltage, and a pulse of sound enters the patient. As this pulse encounters various interfaces of tissue within the patient's body, echoes are reflected back toward the transducer.

When a pulse of ultrasound strikes an interface between two substances, the strength of the reflected echo depends on many factors. A major factor is the mismatch of acoustic impedances of the two substances. If the pulse strikes the interface perpendicularly, the amount reflected will depend on the following equation:

$$R = \frac{Z_1 - Z_2}{Z_1 + Z_2}, \tag{3}$$

where R is reflected energy, Z_1 is acoustic impedance of substance 1, and Z_2 is acoustic impedance of substance 2.

Since the acoustic impedances (Z) of various soft tissues in the body are similar, it becomes evident from equation (3) that only a small amount of energy is reflected at such interfaces. The majority of sound is transmitted through to the next interface:

$$T = 1 - R, \tag{4}$$

where T is transmitted energy and R is reflected energy.

This small amount of reflected energy is necessary in order for enough energy to be transmitted through the patient to visualize structures deep in the body. Ultrasound studies are performed easily through a patient's soft tissue because of this phenomenon.

Why does diagnostic ultrasound encounter such difficulty with ribs, lungs, or bowel air? Why can't structures deep to bone or air be visualized? Equation (2) states that acoustic impedance equals the product of the velocity and density of a substance. Bone and air have acoustic impedances that differ markedly from those of soft tissue. Each has major differences in velocity and density. From equation (3) one can easily predict what will happen at a soft tissue interface in contact with bone or air: there will be a large amount of reflection and very little transmission. Since practically no sound is transmitted through these sites, it is not possible to visualize deeper areas in the patient.

Time Gain Compensation

As a pulse of ultrasound passes through the patient, attenuation of the sound beam occurs at a fairly constant rate in soft tissue. Sound is attenuated at approximately 1 decibel per centimeter traveled for a 1-MHz transducer (1 Db/cm/MHz). If a 5.0-MHz transducer is used, then attenuation in soft tissue approximates 5 Db/cm. More attenuation occurs at higher frequencies, which explains why higher frequency transducers do not penetrate as well as lower frequency transducers.

Echoes returning from deep within the patient are much weaker than surface echoes because of normal body attenuation. If two identical anatomic interfaces are positioned at different levels within the patient, that is, one shallow and one deep, they will not reflect equal echoes back to the transducer. Even though they are similar anatomically, they will appear dramatically different on an ultrasound image because of attenuation. In order to accommodate for this, ultrasound units are constructed with the ability to listen with more sensitivity to the deeper echoes. This occurs through time gain compensation, or TGC.

When the correct TGC is chosen, identical anatomic structures will appear similar to each other, regardless of their depth within the patient. Since a higher frequency experiences more attenuation, the TGC slope must also be higher. Correct assignment of TGC becomes important diagnostically. This is discussed in the Appendix section on enhanced through transmission.

Resolution

The ability to resolve small anatomic structures in close proximity has improved dramatically in recent years. Diagnostic ultrasound requires two types of resolution: axial and lateral.

Axial resolution is the ability to separate two structures situated one in front of the other. For ultrasound, axial resolution is dependent on wavelength (λ) and pulse width. A smaller wavelength yields better axial resolution, so that a higher frequency (smaller wavelength) transducer produces sharper and more useful images. Higher frequency transducers, however, do not penetrate as well as lower frequency transducers. A general rule of thumb is to use the highest frequency transducer that permits adequate penetration of the anatomic area to be examined.

A shorter pulse width also improves axial resolution. Pulse width is affected by the amount of time and strength of the voltage that is applied to a piezoelectric crystal when it acts as a transmitter. A shorter pulse width improves axial resolution. Usual pulse widths are in the range of 1 to 3 μsec.

Lateral resolution is the ability to separate two structures that are side by side. Lateral resolution depends on the width of the ultrasonic beam at different depths within the patient. The diameter of a piezoelectric crystal and the area of its focal zone affect lateral resolution. If an ultrasonic beam is focused, the best lateral resolution is obtained in the focal zone. Correct transducer choice is important when examining anatomic areas at different depths within the patient.

Axial resolution is superior to lateral resolution in diagnostic ultrasound. Best results are obtained in the clinical setting when using axial resolution. Conscious attempts should be made to use axial resolution when scanning.

Reflection

Two major types of reflection occur in a patient and depend on the shape and size of the reflecting surface. Specular reflection occurs when a wave strikes a large smooth interface. The surface must be much larger than the wavelength (λ). If a sound beam strikes an interface perpendicularly, the reflected echo returns to the transducer. If the beam strikes an interface a few degrees off the perpendicular, only a portion of the returning echo will strike the transducer. Since the transducer is a finite size, a reflected echo may miss the transducer completely and not register on the scan. This occurs when a beam strikes an interface far off the perpendicular.

Specular reflectors are the large anatomic boundaries of structures such as the renal capsule, gallbladder wall, blood vessels, diaphragm, and chorionic plate. When a sound beam strikes these interfaces close to the perpendicular, these surfaces will be visualized on a scan. Therefore, it is necessary to scan various anatomic areas at different angles in order to see specular reflectors. An excellent example is the chorionic plate of the placenta. This anatomic structure will be seen only when scanned appropriately and will not be seen when the transducer is not properly aligned. Specular reflectors are the strongest reflectors in the body but are visualized only when scanned correctly.

A second type of reflector is a diffuse, parenchymal, or scattered reflector. It occurs at irregular surfaces or anatomic areas that are smaller in size than the wavelength. Diffuse reflectors differ in two important ways from specular reflectors: they are much weaker than specular reflectors, and their reflected echoes are scattered in all directions so that some returning echoes will always reach the transducer if they are strong enough. These parenchymal echoes arise from various organs of the body, and each organ has a characteristic parenchymal pattern. An example of this is the placenta. When the placenta is anterior, its parenchymal echoes are strong enough to return to the transducer, and the parenchymal pattern of an anterior placenta will be seen in its entirety. Thus, an anterior placenta will have an even parenchymal pattern; whereas its surface, the chorionic plate, which is a specular reflector, will be seen only when the transducer is close to the perpendicular.

When the placenta is situated posteriorly, its ultrasonic presentation will differ according to anterior structures. If amniotic fluid is situated anteriorly, the placental parenchymal pattern will be visualized, since there is only slight attenuation of sound by fluid. Under these circumstances, the weak parenchymal echoes of a posterior placenta will be able to return to the transducer. Note, however, that when the fetus is situated anterior to a posterior placenta, these parenchymal echoes will not be able to reach the transducer because of the high attenuation of sound by the fetus, and the placenta will have a sonolucent appearance. Therefore, a posterior placenta will have a varied ultrasonic appearance.

Critical-Angle Shadowing

When a sound beam strikes a smooth specular interface at an angle other than the perpendicular, more of the energy will be reflected and less will be transmitted through the interface. Eventually, an angle is reached where the amount of reflection increases enough that shadowing will be present. This becomes important clinically at areas such as the top of the urinary bladder. Critical-angle shadowing is manifested in this region with a drop-off in parenchymal echoes of the mid and lower uterine segment. This finding often is misinterpreted as fibroids.

Enhanced Through Transmission

In the discussion of TGC, emphasis was placed on its correct assignment. TGC compensates for the normal attenuation of sound by the body's soft tissue. Fluid-containing structures do not attenuate sound to any significant degree. When a sound beam passes through a fluid-containing structure, the expected attenuation does not occur. If TGC is correctly adjusted for soft tissue, this lack of attenuation is manifested as higher amplitude echoes behind a fluid structure. This enhanced through transmission is diagnostically significant in characterizing the nature of fluid-containing masses.

Reverberation Artifact

When a sound beam strikes a highly reflective surface such as bone or air, most of the energy is reflected back toward the transducer. Since the skin-transducer interface is also highly reflective, this can create a secondary wave, which is transmitted back into the patient. These reverberations, created by highly reflective interfaces, represent the bouncing of sound between the transducer and the highly reflective interface. Reverberation artifacts may cause diagnostic problems if they are not carefully analyzed. Care must be taken to avoid this pitfall when evaluating scans of highly reflective surfaces.

Acoustic Shadowing

Most sound is reflected and very little is transmitted at a bone or air interface. This leads to acoustic shadowing behind such interfaces. When calcified areas in the body are scanned, acoustic shadowing results. Such findings are present in gallstones, renal calculi, teeth within a dermoid, and other pathologic entities. Identification of acoustic shadowing may lead to the correct diagnosis.

B-Scan versus Real Time

Until recently B-scan ultrasound was the major two-dimensional means of imaging. A B-scan, which is similar to a photograph, is a single image of a section through the body. It takes approximately 2 to 5 seconds to produce a B-scan by means of an articulated scanning arm. The images are of high quality and resolution. The major disadvantage is that it is time consuming and cannot evaluate areas in motion.

Real-time ultrasound is similar to a motion picture, but until recent years its image quality and resolution were substandard compared to images produced by B-scan. Improvement in real-time image quality has yielded the advantages of quickness of scan, visualization of motion, and flexibility of scanning approach—features that far outweigh the advantages of B-scanning. B-scanners now are generally being replaced by high-resolution real-time scanners.

Real-time scanners basically are of two types: mechanical scanners and array system. Each has advantages and disadvantages. Real-time scanners generate individual images so quickly that the eye perceives a motion picture as the scanner moves over the patient.

Selected Readings

Sample, W. F., and Erikson, K. Basic principles of diagnostic ultrasound. In *Diagnostic ultrasound: text and cases,* eds. D. A. Sarti and W. F. Sample. Boston: G.K. Hall, 1980.

McDicken, W. N. *Diagnostic ultrasonics.* New York: John Wiley & Sons, 1975.

Wells, P. N. T. *Physical principles of ultrasonic diagnosis.* Kingston, Ontario: Ultramedison, 1976.

CASES

Sound-Tissue Interactions

Figure 322 represents a phantom developed by Dr. Nabil F. Maklad and Dr. Jonathan Ophir at the University of Kansas Medical Center, Kansas City, Kansas. The background material within the phantom has acoustic properties similar to those of liver tissue. Inserted within the phantom are various circular materials of varying size with different acoustic properties. In the upper row are a series of 1.6-cm diameter substances; in the lower row 0.6-cm diameter structures are interposed. In Sections A and B of the phantom the material has a decreased attenuation. In addition, in section A the material is surrounded by a membrane across which a velocity change occurs. The velocity of sound in the background material is 1540 meters per second whereas the velocity of sound within the membrane is 2000 meters per second. In section C of the phantom the material has an increase of 30% in attenuation and in section B of the phantom the material has an increase of 200% in attenuation without any change in velocity of the sound.

In section A of the phantom, where velocity changes occur at the membrane, its shadowing effects are observed.

In area B of the phantom, where no velocity changes take place, only the enhancement of the sound beyond the region is appreciated; this is related to the lower attenuation through the area. In section C of the phantom, the material causing the increased attenuation can be visualized, as well as the deeper shadowing effects related to the attenuation. In contrast, in region D of the phantom, the actual material causing the attenuation cannot be visualized; however, the shadowing effects of the attenuation are appreciated.

A clinical example of velocity changes is provided in figure 323. This longitu-

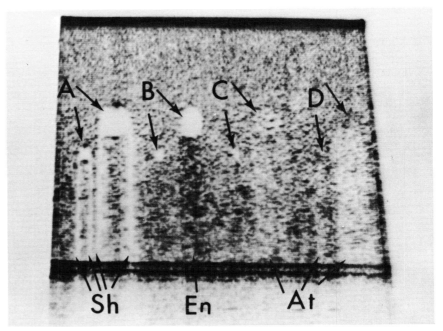

Fig. 322

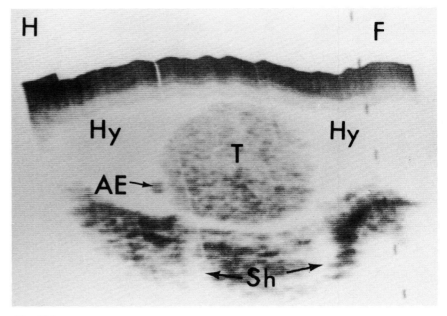

Fig. 323

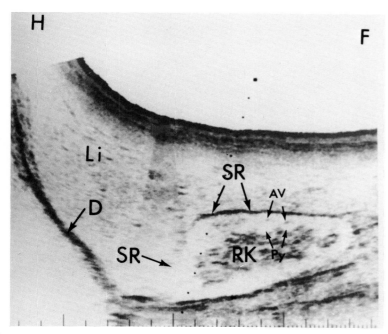

Fig. 324

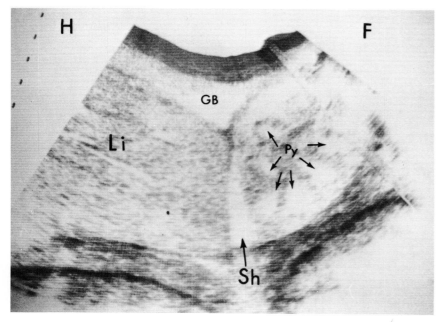

Fig. 325

dinal scan of a scrotum shows a testicle surrounded by a hydrocele. The difference in velocities in the two materials leads to the shadowing effects. Figures 324 and 325 represent clinical examples of the inclination dependence of specular reflectors. The interface between the kidney and the liver represents a specular reflector. It is, however, variable in contour so that only when the scanning beam is pointed relatively perpendicular to the interface is the tissue plane recorded. The tissue plane frequently is lost in the upper pole of the kidney, since the reflections that occur never return to the transducer. Instead, they are reflected back to an area on the skin surface, where the transducer is not present, and are not recorded.

In figure 325 the beneficial effects of the inability to see specular reflectors when they are parallel or inclined to the sound beam is demonstrated by the ability to differentiate the pyramids of the kidney from the surrounding cortex. Generally, when the scanning beam is kept perpendicular to the renal capsule, the interfaces within the pyramids are parallel or sufficiently inclined in relation to the sound beam so that they are not recorded. In contrast, the rather haphazardly organized interfaces within the renal cortex, many of which are diffuse reflectors, are recorded regardless of the inclination of the beam. A shadowing effect is also demonstrated secondary to the velocity changes that occur at the liver and gallbladder renal interfaces.

AE	=	Appendix epididymis
At	=	Attenuation
AV	=	Arcuate vessels
D	=	Diaphragm
En	=	Enhancement
F	=	Feet
GB	=	Gallbladder
H	=	Head
Hy	=	Hydrocele
Li	=	Liver
Py	=	Renal pyramids
RK	=	Right kidney
Sh	=	Shadowing
SR	=	Specular reflector
T	=	Testis

Sound-Tissue Interactions Related to Velocity Changes I.

In this set of clinical examples, the potentially detrimental effects of shadowing related to velocity changes are illustrated. In figure 326 the amniotic fluid surrounding the fetal head and extremities represents interfaces with major velocity changes. Shadows occur at the edges of these curvilinear surfaces and are related to critical-angle phenomena. The shadowed area deep to the edges may make localization of the placenta difficult. In many instances, moving the position of the mother in order to change the position of the fetal head is necessary in order to determine the exact location of the placenta in relationship to the endocervical canal.

In figure 327 the shadowing effect of the bladder-uterine interface in this longitudinal scan of a postpartum mother prevents visualization of the acoustic texture of the uterus in this region. Since this area is the region where cesarean sections are performed and is susceptible to various complications, such as hematoma or abscess, the sound beam must be manipulated to avoid this interface and shadowing effect.

Figure 328 represents a common shadowing effect related to velocity changes. At the edges of the gallbladder and, most importantly, near the neck where multiple surfaces created by the spiral valves are present, shadowing on the basis of critical-angle or refractive phenomena can occur. These shadows can mimic stones unless this normal variant is appreciated. In these situations movement of the patient to try to alter the orientation of the sound beam, and therefore the shadowing, is necessary before stones can be excluded.

A similar situation is created when the gallbladder is folded upon itself or has an incomplete septation such as is demonstrated in figure 329. The velocity change occurring at the bile-infolding interface can lead to a shadow which simulates a calculus. Generally, the movement of the patient into various positions will cause an unfolding of the gallbladder, and this normal variant will be recognized.

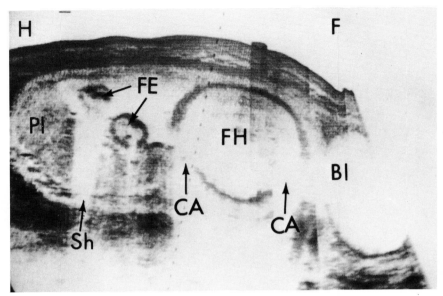

Fig. 326

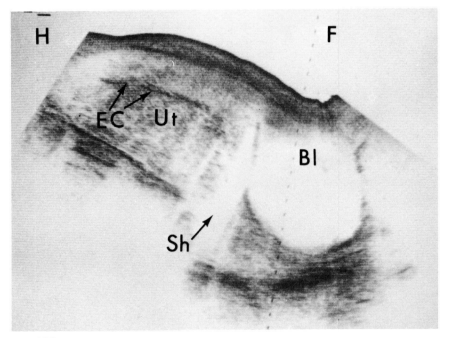

Fig. 327

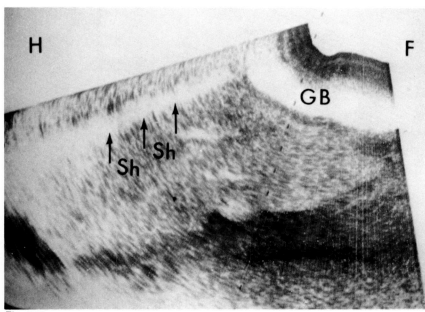

Fig. 328

Bl	=	Bladder
CA	=	Critical angle
EC	=	Endometrial canal
F	=	Foot
FE	=	Fetal extremities
FHe	=	Fetal head
GB	=	Gallbladder
H	=	Head
In	=	Infolding
Li	=	Liver
Pl	=	Placenta
Sh	=	Shadowing
Ut	=	Uterus

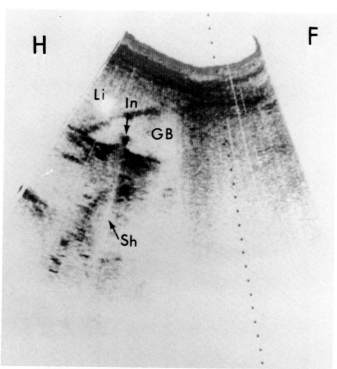

Fig. 329

Sound-Tissue Interactions Related to Velocity Changes II.

The shadowing effects related to velocity changes at curvilinear specular interfaces may provide differentially diagnostic information. In figure 330 an amebic abscess is present within the liver. The lower attenuation of the abscess, in spite of the internal solid elements, is indicated by the enhancement in the deeper region of the liver. The presence of its shadowing also indicates that velocity changes are occurring. The importance of the shadowing effects of various types of masses may be related to wall characteristics that could have differential diagnostic significance. Considerably more work in this area is necessary to determine the exact nature of this differential diagnostic information.

In figure 331 a limited high-resolution scan using a high-frequency real-time system demonstrates two shadowing effects relating to velocity changes in the region of the common carotid artery. The shadowing effects allow the sonographer actually to visualize the thickness of the carotid wall, which cannot be visualized by means of acoustic impedance differences alone.

An important differentially diagnostic aspect of shadowing related to velocity changes frequently is observed in the gallbladder area. A gallbladder filled with stone may be difficult to outline. The shadowing effects related to what are probably velocity changes at the stone interfaces, however, lead to a type of shadowing that is distinctly different from the gas-containing nearby duodenum (fig. 332). In the case of the former, the shadowing has little reverberation or noise within it. In contrast, at the air interface of the duodenum, which is a total reflector returning the sound to the transducer, a series of reverberation and ring-

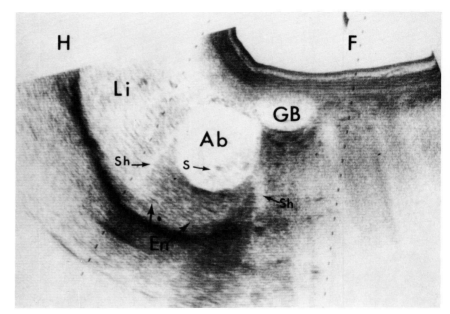

Fig. 330

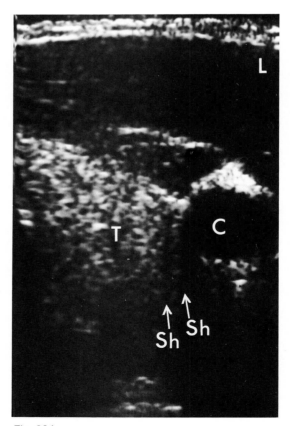

Fig. 331

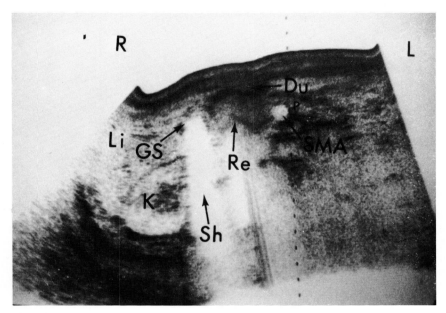

Fig. 332

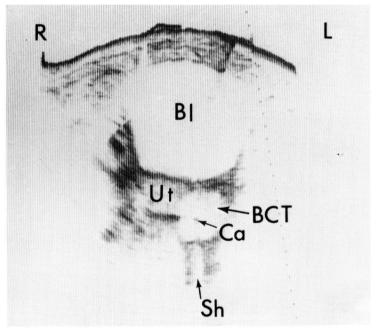

Fig. 333

down artifacts leading to a noisy or "dirty" type of shadowing is observed. Therefore, the different types of shadowing resulting from the different interreactions of the sound beam allow proper identification of an abnormal gallbladder even though the gallbladder itself is not visualized.

Figure 333 illustrates a relatively nonspecific appearing adnexal mass, which could have an extensive differential diagnosis. The presence of an interface within the mass, however, is related to a significant velocity change resulting in shadowing and suggests the presence of calcification. This places the mass in a more limited differentially diagnostic grouping that includes benign cystic teratoma which was proven at surgery.

Ab = Abscess
BCT = Benign cystic teratoma
Bl = Bladder
C   = Common cartoid artery
Ca = Calcium
Du = Duodenum
En = Enhancement
F   = Foot
GB = Gallbladder
GS = Gallstone
H   = Head
K   = Kidney
L   = Left
Li = Liver
P   = Pancreas
R   = Right
Re = Reverberation
S   = Solid elements
Sh = Shadowing
SMA = Superior mesenteric artery
T   = Thyroid
Ut = Uterus

Total Ultrasonic Reflectors

The major complete reflector within the body represents air. In addition to the shadowing effect, the very strong reflections lead to a series of reverberation and ring-down artifacts. In figure 334, the typical appearance of artifacts associated with a total reflector is seen. In this case, a linear cap of gas in the stomach overlying the pancreas is illustrated. Each reverberation has regular periodic qualities and is associated with a tail ring-down artifact. Each subsequent reverberation is narrower, thinner, and associated with a smaller ring-down tail.

Figure 335 illustrates an additional feature of a reverberation artifact. Since it represents the bouncing back and forth between two surfaces, the configuration of the reverberation is the summation effect of the configuration of the two interfaces. In this case, the configurations of the skin and the linear cap of gas are different; as a result, the configuration of the reverberation is significantly different from that of the total reflector. The source of the reverberation is still easily identified by the associated shadowing and the tail of ring down.

When a gas pocket is spherical in shape, the total reflection is inclined and never returns to the transducer, leading to a clean type of shadowing (fig. 336). This most frequently occurs in the small bubble of gas in the duodenal bulb and can mimic the clean shadowing resulting from velocity changes in an abnormal gallbladder. Therefore, when the diagnosis of an abnormal gallbladder, based on shadowing related to velocity changes, is entertained, the duodenum must be specifically identified.

In general, artifacts related to total reflectors are easily identified, but they still may cause problems in scan interpretation. In figure 337, the artifacts associated with the total reflectors make determination of the extent of the aneurysm difficult. If the gas pockets were more generalized, the aneurysm could be entirely obscured.

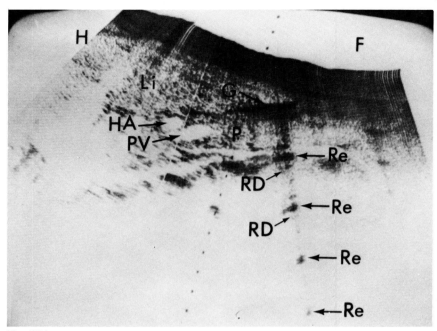

Fig. 334

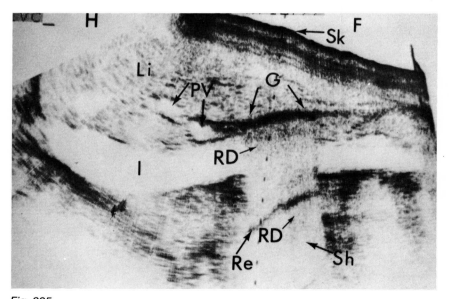

Fig. 335

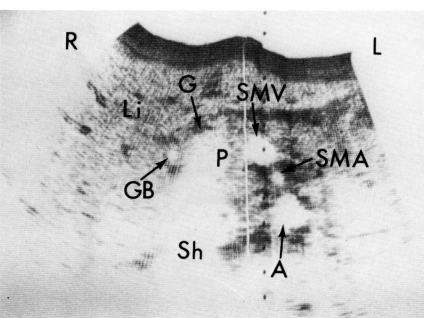

Fig. 336

A	=	Aorta
An	=	Aneurysm
Co	=	Colon
F	=	Foot
G	=	Gas
GB	=	Gallbladder
H	=	Head
HA	=	Hepatic artery
I	=	Inferior vena cava
L	=	Left
Li	=	Liver
P	=	Pancreas
PV	=	Portal vein
R	=	Right
RD	=	Ring down
Re	=	Reverberation
Sh	=	Shadowing
Sk	=	Skin
SMA	=	Superior mesenteric artery
SMV	=	Superior mesenteric vein
St	=	Stomach

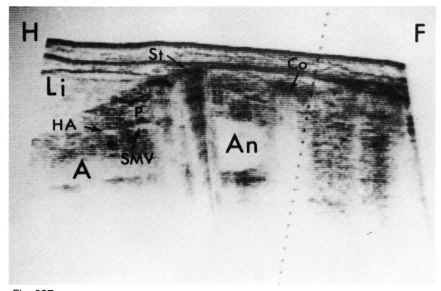

Fig. 337

Total Sound Reflectors

In some cases, the reverberation phenomena created by total reflectors are more difficult to recognize. In figures 338 and 339 the transverse and longitudinal scans of a patient being evaluated for pancreatic disease are provided. A flat cap of gas within the duodenal bulb has resulted in a single reverberation artifact which mimics a true, more deeply situated interface. The resulting through transmission sign is seemingly satisfied, and a mass is misinterpreted in the pancreatic region. The different inclination of the reverberation in figure 339 that results from the differing configurations of the skin and gas pocket further confuses the issue. These types of reverberative phenomena usually can be recognized if multiple scanning approaches are directed at the same interface. Different types of reverberative phenomena usually can be elicited and will allow proper recognition.

Another place where phenomena reverberating off total reflectors frequently occur is in the pelvis. The fluid-filled bladder allows a path of decreased attenuation for such a reverberation even if the total reflecting surface is deep within the pelvis. The apparent mass effect created by reverberation off the gas in the rectal sigmoid portion of the colon passing beneath the adnexa is shown in figure 340. Since the reverberation was associated with very little ring-down noise, a cystic-appearing mass with apparent through transmission was simulated. The apparent through transmission, however, represents the reverberation plus its accompanying ring-down noise.

If the reverberation artifact from gas beneath the bladder is associated with a large amount of noise, a solid-appearing mass within the pelvis can be simulated, as demonstrated in figure 341. The mass in this case mimics an enlarged uterus adjacent to an adnexal fluid collection. Careful questioning of the patient, however, revealed that the uterus had been removed some years ago and led to alternative scanning approaches that demonstrated the artifactual nature of the mass.

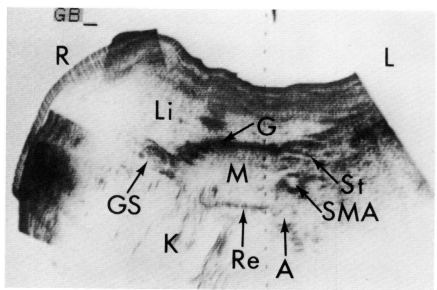

Fig. 338

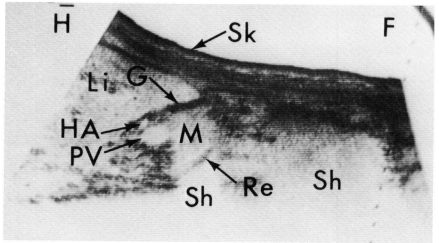

Fig. 339

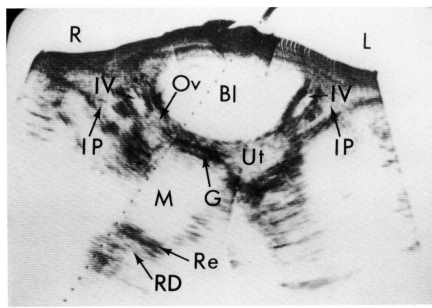

Fig. 340

A   = Aorta
Bl   = Bladder
F   = Foot
Fl   = Fluid
G   = Gas
GS   = Gallstone
H   = Head
HA   = Hepatic artery
IP   = Iliopsoas muscle
IV   = Iliac vessels
K   = Kidney
L   = Left
Li   = Liver
M   = Mass
Ov   = Ovary
PV   = Portal vein
R   = Right
RD   = Ring down
Re   = Reverberation
Sh   = Shadowing
Sk   = Skin
SMA = Superior mesenteric artery
St   = Stomach
Ut   = Uterus

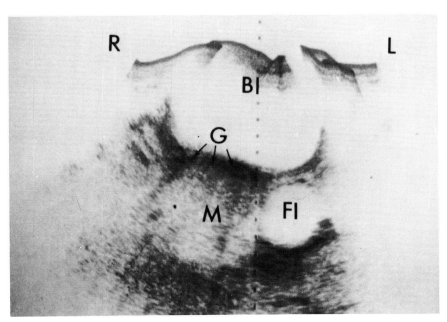

Fig. 341

TGC and
Effects of Areas of
Diminished Attenuation

The time gain compensation curve of the contact B scanner compensates for the average attenuation of tissues. The effects on the ultrasound image of an intervening area of diminished attenuation have certain characteristics which are basic to cyst-solid determinations. In figure 342, the classical differences between a cystic and solid lesion are demonstrated. In this instance there was no velocity change across the interfaces, and therefore, shadowing effects related to refractive or critical-angle phenomena are not observed. Nevertheless, fluid areas of lower attenuation are associated with sharp posterior walls and apparent enhancement of the underlying echo amplitude.

To demonstrate enhancement, however, reflecting surfaces must be beneath the area of decreased attenuation that allows this phenomenon to be observed. In figure 343, two amebic abscesses are present within the liver. The more superficial abscess in the left lobe is associated with shadowing related to velocity changes at the edges as well as enhancement effects related to the lower attenuation demonstrated in the deeper retroperitoneal tissues. The even larger abscess in the deep right lobe abuts directly on the diaphragm-air interface which does not allow the enhancement to be observed, since the interface represents a total reflector.

In some regions of the body, such as the pelvis, even though a normal fluid collection is present for comparison (bladder), total reflectors, such as bowel gas or bone, prevent the enhancement phenomenon from being observed (fig. 344). For cyst-solid differentiation, other features must be sought, such as the relative anterior ring-down phenomenon and the presence of reflections from internal solid components. In this case the different reflectivity of the solid components is readily visible in this complex benign cystic teratoma.

The enhancement phenomenon associated with lower attenuating regions (usually fluid) is still, however, the most reliable sign of a lower attenuator. Therefore, when a mass meets all of the

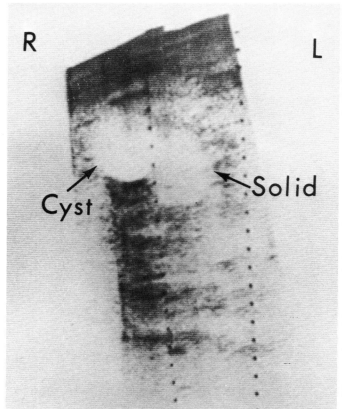

Fig. 342

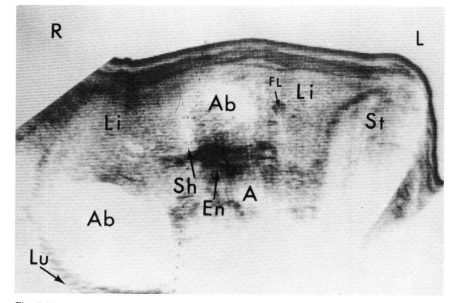

Fig. 343

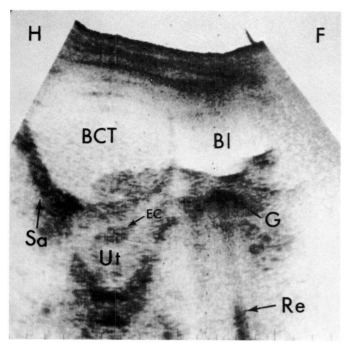

Fig. 344

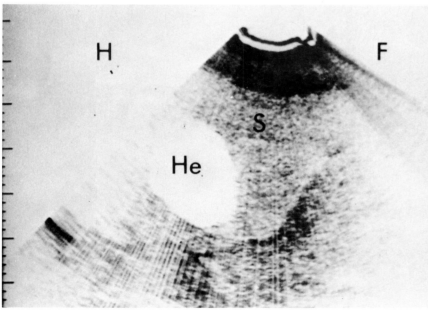

Fig. 345

other criteria of a lower attenuator, such as smooth margins or absence of internal echoes, the absence of enhancement where sufficient tissue is present deep to the area is still the most reliable sign that the mass is not a fluid. This is demonstrated by the clotted hematoma within the spleen in figure 345, which demonstrates all of the characteristics of a fluid mass, with the exception of the enhancement phenomenon. Sufficient splenic tissue and retroperitoneal structures are present deep to the mass, so that enhancement should have occurred if it were, in fact, fluid in nature.

A	= Aorta
Ab	= Abscess
BCT	= Benign cystic teratoma
Bl	= Bladder
EC	= Endometrial canal
En	= Enhancement
F	= Foot
FL	= Falciform ligament
G	= Gas
H	= Head
He	= Hematoma
L	= Left
Li	= Liver
Lu	= Lung
R	= Right
Re	= Reverberation
S	= Spleen
Sa	= Sacrum
Sh	= Shadowing
St	= Stomach
Ut	= Uterus

Artifacts Associated with Areas of Low Attenuation

Interposed regions of low attenuation are associated with a number of artifacts. The acoustic impedance differences at the junction of an average and a low-attenuating tissue usually are substantial and generate relatively strong reflections. When the region of low attenuation is, therefore, close to the transducer, a series of reverberation and ring-down artifacts can be generated within the low-attenuating area. These regions have been recognized in ultrasound as the echoes in the near side of the fluid region (figure 346) and usually are easily identified. However, when the region of low attenuation occurs very superficially, the noise and ring-down phenomena, particularly if the gain settings are somewhat high, can totally obscure the region unless careful attention is paid to underlying enhancement. A typical clinical example is illustrated in figure 347, in which a very superficial renal cyst easily could be missed.

More deeply situated regions of diminished attenuation also can lead to artifacts if there is a nearby strong reflecting surface. A common place for such an artifact to occur is in a cystic or fluid mass within the liver adjacent to the diaphragm. Reverberation artifacts result and give the apparent appearance of a similar mass on the other side of the diaphragm, as indicated in figure 348.

An experimental situation simulating this phenomenon is demonstrated in figure 349. A water bath containing a balloon filled with water is placed midway along the ultrasound beam but adjacent to the highly reflective water-bath wall. While the sound beam is insonating the water-bath wall at an inclination, reflections are set up which reverberate off the balloon and simulate a similarly configured mass in the air outside of the container. This experiment was conducted by Fred Gardner, one of our technicians at the University of California School of Medicine, Los Angeles, California.

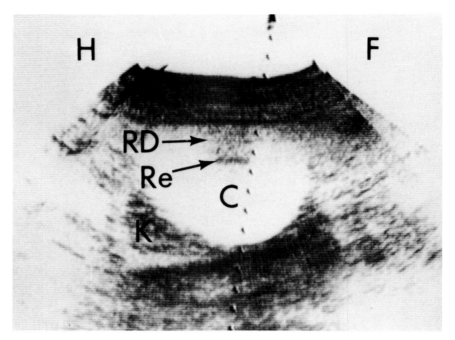

Fig. 346

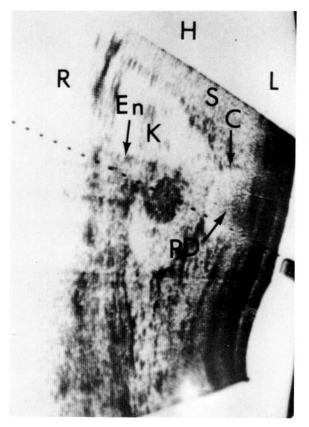

Fig. 347

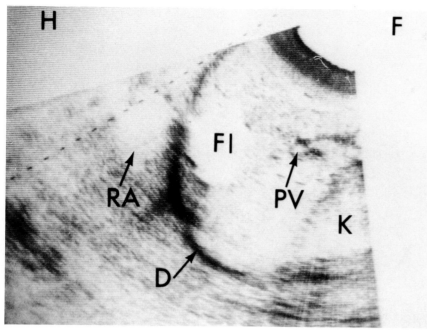

B	=	Balloon
C	=	Cyst
D	=	Diaphragm
En	=	Enhancement
F	=	Foot
FI	=	Fluid
H	=	Head
K	=	Kidney
L	=	Left
PV	=	Portal vein
R	=	Right
RA	=	Reverberation artifact
RD	=	Ring down
Re	=	Reverberation
S	=	Spleen

Fig. 348

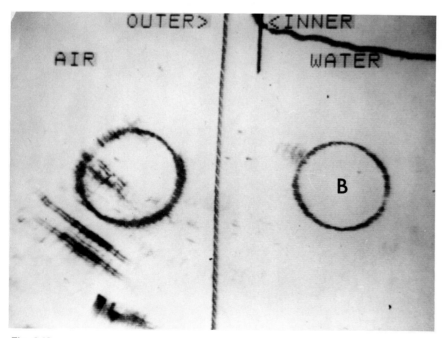

Fig. 349

Effects of Areas of Diminished Attenuation

The comparison of the acoustic textures of various organs has become an important part of ultrasonography. In general, the relative reflectivity of various organs compared at the same depth within the body can be a reliable indicator of certain diseases. If an area of diminished attenuation is present between the transducer and one of the tissues, however, fallacious overamplification of the acoustic texture will occur. If this is not recognized, the appearance of an abnormal organ texture can be simulated. A typical example is illustrated in figures 350 and 351. Normally the amplitude of echoes arising from the renal cortex is slightly less than that of the liver. In figure 350, however, the texture comparison is made with the lower-attenuating gallbladder intervening between the sound beam and the kidney. The apparently abnormal, greater-amplitude echoes of the renal parenchyma, as compared to the liver, suggest some form of generalized renal disease. In figure 351, however, the patient has been moved into the decubitus position, throwing the lower-attenuating gallbladder out of the field of comparison. As a result, a more appropriate relative amplitude texture comparison between the kidney and liver can be made.

Similarly, difficulty in recognizing certain components of a gestation may result from the intervening amniotic fluid, as demonstrated in figures 352 and 353. In figure 352, because of the overamplification resulting from the intervening amniotic fluid as well as from an inappropriately high gain setting, it is impossible to tell whether the thickened posterior wall of the gestation represents a placental tongue or a uterine contraction. In figure 353 the gain settings and time gain compensation have been readjusted, so that the proper acoustic texture of the posterior gestational wall can be analyzed. The texture is seen to be different from that of the anterior placenta and, therefore, identified as a uterine contraction.

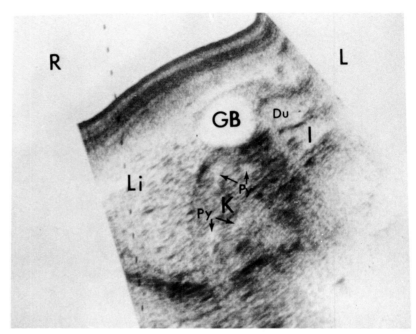

Fig. 350

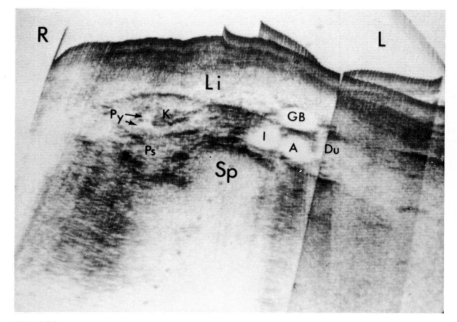

Fig. 351

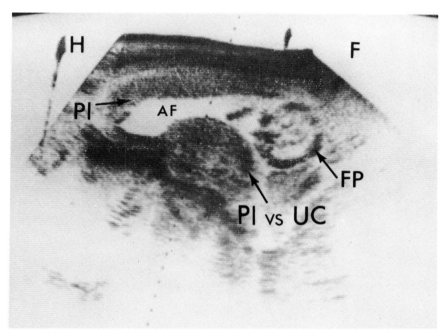

Fig. 352

A	=	Aorta
AF	=	Amniotic fluid
Du	=	Duodenum
F	=	Foot
FH	=	Fetal head
FP	=	Fetal parts
GB	=	Gallbladder
H	=	Head
I	=	Inferior vena cava
K	=	Kidney
L	=	Left
Li	=	Liver
Pl	=	Placenta
Pl vs UC	=	Placenta vs uterine contractions
Ps	=	Psoas muscle
Py	=	Renal pyramids
R	=	Right
Sp	=	Spine
UC	=	Uterine contraction

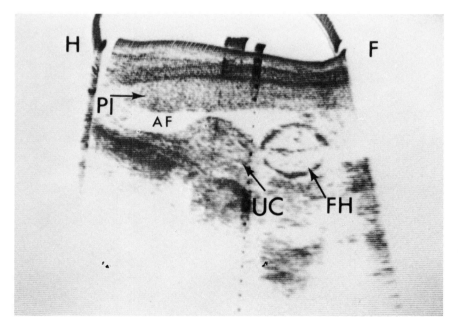

Fig. 353

Effects of Areas of Increased Attenuation I.

A number of areas of increased attenuation occur normally and pathologically within the body. In normal cases, if the resulting phenomena of the increased attenuation are not appreciated, an incorrect diagnosis can be made. A common high attenuator within the upper abdomen is the falciform ligament, accompanied by its extension within the liver, the ligamentum teres. This represents a dense fibrous band which is highly attenuative of the ultrasound beam. As a result, the underlying ultrasonic textures are of a lower amplitude than usual. The effects of this phenomenon are illustrated in figure 354. The head of the pancreas is identified precisely by anatomic landmarks that include the gallbladder, duodenum, common bile duct, superior mesenteric vein, and superior mesenteric artery. In addition, the scanning around the falciform ligament has provided through transmission, so that the prevertebral vessels, the crus of the diaphragm, and the anterior surface of the spine are visualized. Due to the attenuation process in the falciform ligament, the acoustic texture and relative amplitude of the pancreas are not, however, properly registered. As a result, a pancreatic abnormality might be suspected if the effects of the falciform ligament are not realized.

A similar situation is created by scars in the skin and subcutaneous tissues. These often are difficult to see, yet their effects on the attenuation of the sound and the underlying acoustic texture are dramatic. In figure 355, a small scar in the subcutaneous tissues has caused a dramatic attenuation and shadowing effect which has resulted in a wide area of abnormal texture throughout the underlying liver. In figure 356, the patient has been rescanned, and the scar area was avoided during the scanning process. The more normal hepatic acoustic texture, as well as the clear visualization of interhepatic vascular anatomy, is appreciated. For this reason, when scanning portions of the body where scars are likely to occur, it is best to hold the transducer between the

thumb and index finger and slide the third, fourth, and fifth digits in contact across the skin in order to palpate the scar.

Figure 357 represents an excellent example of the combined effects of the

presence of areas of increased and decreased attenuation. In this transverse scan of a gestational uterus, a remarkable difference in the acoustic texture of the placenta is appreciated. The normal acoustic texture of the placenta is ap-

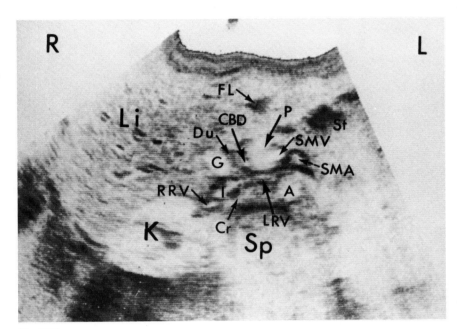

Fig. 354

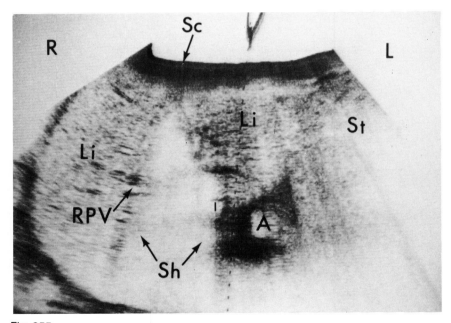

Fig. 355

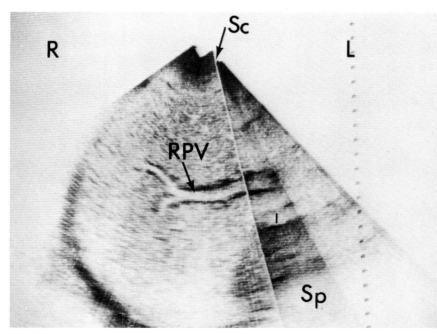

Fig. 356

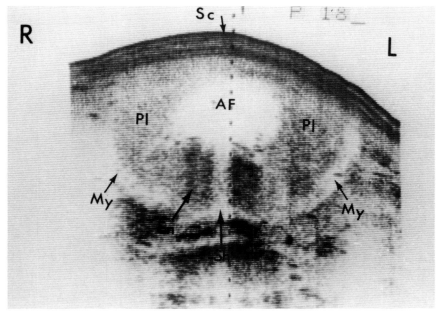

Fig. 357

section scar. Finally, the placental texture of the left side of the uterus is noted to be slightly higher in amplitude than that of the right, with no intervening fluid. This demonstrates the effect of the scanning speed on the acoustic texture in analog systems. Since most analog systems use a peak detection system, the actual amplitudes of the reflections received from an area are subject to a sampling error. The faster the sonographer scans, the less likely the optimal reflection from that area will be achieved. Therefore, when comparing various textures with analog systems, a constant scanning speed is required.

A	=	Aorta
AF	=	Amniotic fluid
CBD	=	Common bile duct
Cr	=	Crus of the diaphragm
Du	=	Duodenum
En	=	Enhancement
FL	=	Falciform ligament
G	=	Gallbladder
I	=	Inferior vena cava
K	=	Kidney
L	=	Left
Li	=	Liver
LRV	=	Left renal vein
My	=	Myometrium
P	=	Pancreas
Pl	=	Placenta
R	=	Right
RPV	=	Right portal vein
RRV	=	Right renal vein
Sc	=	Scar
Sh	=	Shadowing
SMA	=	Superior mesenteric artery
SMV	=	Superior mesenteric vein
Sp	=	Spine
St	=	Stomach

preciated on the right side of the uterus. A higher amplitude acoustic texture is noted in the region deep to the amniotic fluid. This has resulted from an inappropriate amplification related to the standard time gain compensation. In addition, a shadowed area of decreased placental texture is noted within this region. It is secondary to the attenuation resulting from a superficial cesarean-

Effects of Areas of Increased Attenuation II.

The increased attenuation process is an important sign of pathology. Depending upon the region of the body, however, the appreciation of the increased attenuation may be difficult. Furthermore, the entire path of the sound beam must be appreciated if this sign is to be used as an indicator of disease.

A common entity which may only be recognized by an area of increased attenuation is the presence of a benign cystic teratoma within the pelvis. Figure 358 demonstrates, in the left adnexal region, an area of increased attenuation which is associated with a deformity of the bladder wall. This could be related to a large gassy area within the colon; however, the rectosigmoid region is identified on the opposite side of the pelvis. Figure 359 demonstrates in another case how the posterior wall of a highly attenuative mass may still be demonstrated by appropriate changes in the gain settings.

Another area where increased attenuation is associated with disease is in cirrhosis of the liver. In figure 360, a small liver surrounded by ascitic fluid should normally have a consistent strong acoustic texture. This liver, however, has been markedly scarred from the cirrhotic process, and the decreased texture in the deeper parts of the liver, a result of the attenuation process, can be appreciated. In the deeper regions of the liver, underlying the gallbladder which counteracts this attenuation by the lower attenuation of the bile, the two processes offset one another and give rise to an apparently normal liver texture.

Figure 361 is also a patient with cirrhosis and ascites. The sections of the liver and spleen are similar in size and surrounded by similar amounts of ascites. Therefore, the decreased attenuation seen in the deeper areas of the liver is real and aids in the differential diagnosis of the ascites.

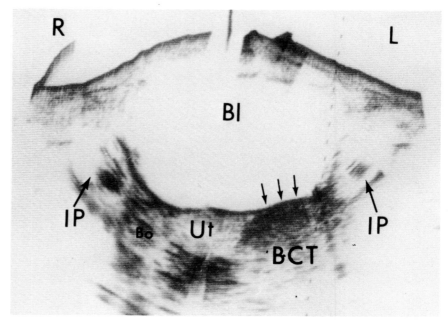

Fig. 358

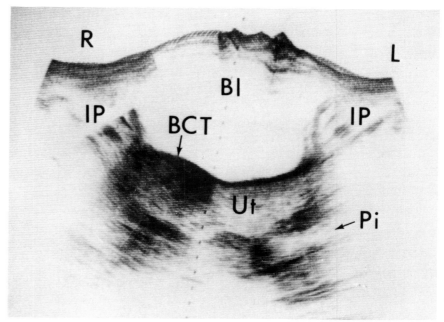

Fig. 359

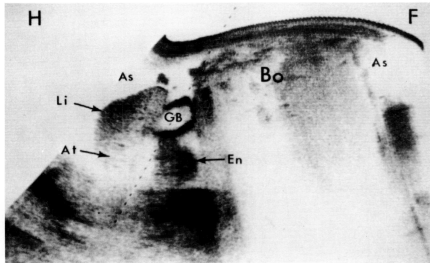

Fig. 360

A	=	Aorta
Arrows	=	Bladder wall indentation
As	=	Ascites
At	=	Attenuation
BCT	=	Benign cystic teratoma
Bl	=	Bladder
Bo	=	Bowel
En	=	Enhancement
F	=	Foot
GB	=	Gallbladder
H	=	Head
I	=	Inferior vena cava
IP	=	Iliopsoas muscle
K	=	Kidney
L	=	Left
Li	=	Liver
Pi	=	Piriformis muscle
Ps	=	Psoas muscle
R	=	Right
S	=	Spleen
Sp	=	Spine
Ut	=	Uterus

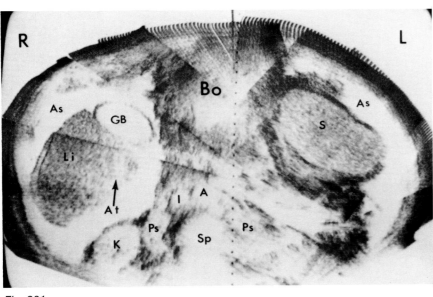

Fig. 361

Effects of Beamwidth

Since the beamwidth characteristics of a transducer lead to the writing of the echo as a line rather than a dot, the wall characteristics of a mass should be analyzed with the better resolving axial resolution of the system. In figure 362, a large cystic mass anterior to the uterus is identified. Portions of its wall, however, are imaged with the lateral resolving capabilities of the beam leading to linear projections into the cyst. These can be mistaken for solid components and thus lead to misinterpretation. The proper scanning technique for such a large cystic mass is demonstrated in figures 363–365. Each segment of the wall is scanned with the axial resolution of the system by keeping the scanning path perpendicular to the wall contour. The beamwidth artifacts are no longer visualized, and the proper conclusion of a simple fluid area is made.

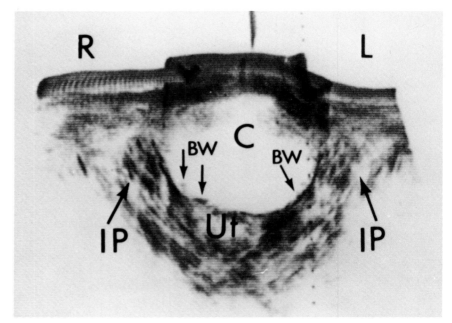

Fig. 362

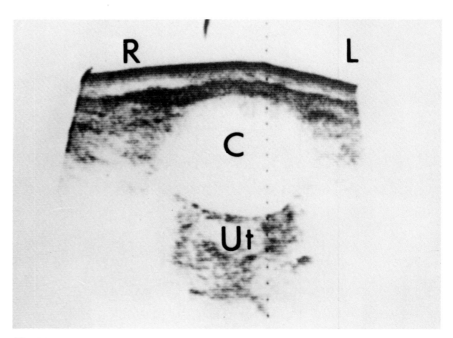

Fig. 363

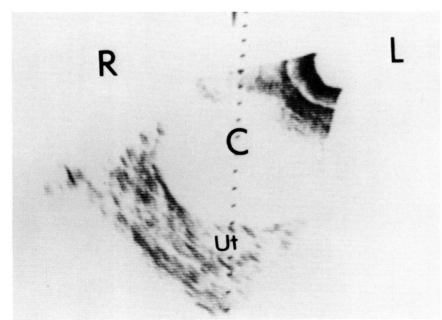

BW = Beamwidth artifacts
C = Cyst
Ip = Iliopsoas muscle
L = Left
R = Right
Ut = Uterus

Fig. 364

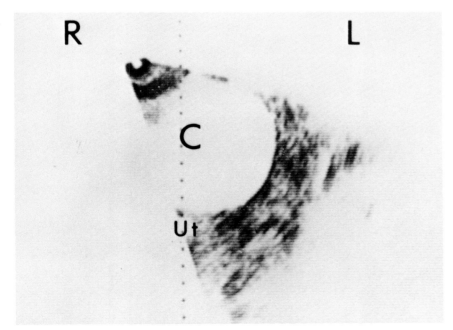

Fig. 365

Effects of Compression Curve Assignment

With analog scan converter systems, the compression curve assignment is critical to high-quality scans. The appropriate gray scale mapping, gain settings, and scanning technique lead to the type of spatial and contrast resolution indicated by figure 366. In this longitudinal scan of the liver, intricate detail of the vascular anatomy is seen. A relatively homogeneous acoustic texture pattern is also possible, in spite of the beam intensity profile effects. In addition, the echo amplitude differences between the kidney and the liver can be appreciated. Only with this type of technique can subtle, solid abnormalities and acoustic texture, such as those seen with a slightly more reflective metastasis, be appreciated (fig. 367).

Similarly, the variety of acoustic textures and gray tones within the gestational uterus (fig. 368) requires proper compression curve assignment, machine setup, and scanning technique. Only then can subtle differences in acoustic texture indicating such abnormalities as a myoma in conjunction with a gestation (fig. 369) be recognized.

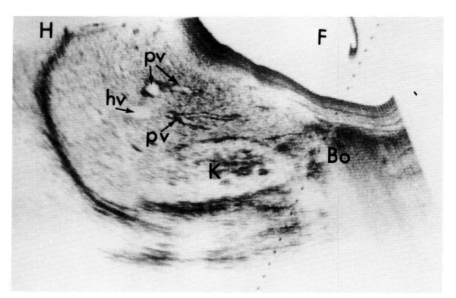

Fig. 366

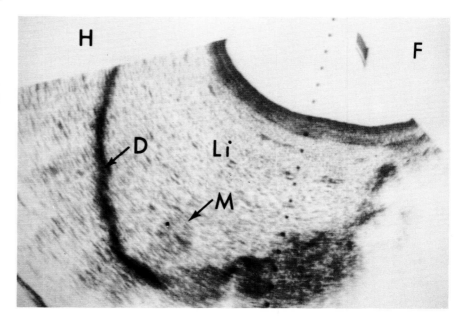

Fig. 367

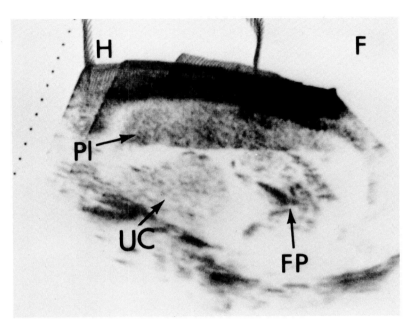

Fig. 368

AF = Amniotic fluid
Bo = Bowel
D   = Diaphragm
F   = Foot
FP = Fetal parts
H   = Head
hv = Hepatic vein
IP = Iliopsoas muscle
K   = Kidney
L   = Left
Li = Liver
M   = Metastases
My = Myometrium
Myo = Myoma
Pl = Placenta
pv = Portal vein
R   = Right
UC = Uterine contraction

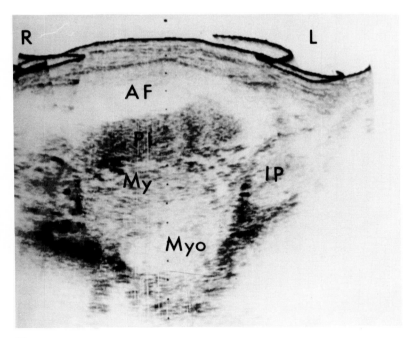

Fig. 369

The following figures have been reproduced in this text with the permission of the editors and publishers of their respective book or journal:
Figures 191–193, 195, 196, 198, 199, 201, 230, 340: Sample, W. F. Normal anatomy of the female pelvis: computed tomography and ultrasonography. In *Clinics in diagnostic ultrasound 2.* New York: Churchill Livingstone, 1979, pp. 191–205.

Figures 352, 353: Sample, W. F. The unsoftened portion of the uterus: a pitfall in gray scale ultrasound studies during midtrimester pregnancy. *Radiology* 126:227–230, 1978.

Index